Clinical implications of
laboratory tests

Clinical implications of laboratory tests

SARKO M. TILKIAN, M.D.

Director of Medical Education, Northridge Hospital, Northridge, Calif.;
Staff Physician, Northridge Hospital, Northridge, Calif.;
Valley Presbyterian Hospital, Van Nuys, Calif.;
Granada Hills Hospital, Granada Hills, Calif.

MARY H. CONOVER, R.N., B.S.N.Ed.

Instructor in Continuing Education, West Park Hospital, Canoga Park, Calif., and
San Fernando Hospital, San Fernando, Calif.; formerly Instructor in Electrocardiography
and CCU Nursing at California State University, Northridge, Calif., and College of the
Canyons, Valencia, Calif.; Instructor in basic and advanced arrhythmia courses,
Los Angeles, Calif.

CONTRIBUTOR

ARA G. TILKIAN, M.D.

Fellow in Cardiology, Stanford University Hospital, Stanford, Calif.

with 42 illustrations

The C. V. Mosby Company

Saint Louis   1975

Library of Congress Cataloging in Publication Data

Tilkian, Sarko M   1936-
    Clinical implications of laboratory tests.

    Bibliography: p.
    Includes index.
    1. Medicine, Clinical.   2. Diagnosis.
I. Conover, Mary H., joint author.   II. Title.
[DNLM: 1. Diagnosis, Laboratory.   QY4   T573c]
RB37.T54   616.07'5   75-15951
ISBN 0-8016-4961-7

TS/M/M   9   8   7   6   5

Preface

This book is designed for persons in the nursing and allied health professions who need a concise reference and comprehensive guide to the clinical significance of laboratory tests. It is our intention to bridge the gap between the voluminous clinical pathology textbooks and the handbooks that merely list the conditions associated with abnormal laboratory results.

The routine laboratory screening panel discussed in Unit One suggests one or several possible disease entities that could be suspected when a particular laboratory test or combination of laboratory tests is abnormal. The table provided at the end of Unit One will guide the reader to the page in Unit Two where further discussion of the suspected disease entity and additional laboratory tests can be found that will help confirm the diagnosis.

In Unit Two the anatomy and physiology of the system involved will be discussed briefly before the specific laboratory tests so that the rationale behind the test and the nomenclature and limitations of the specific tests may be better understood. Pathophysiology is presented when it is necessary for the understanding of terminology. The laboratory tests related to the organ system will then be described, and followed, in most chapters, by their use in the clinical setting. Finally, specific disease entities will be discussed with emphasis on laboratory tests and the differential diagnosis. The purpose of this approach is to avoid "tunnel vision" in the interpretation of laboratory tests. It is common to find that a test, although reported to be within "normal" range, is significantly aberrant when evaluated in relation to the other parameters. In some chapters, disease entities are too numerous for separate discussion and are mentioned therefore with the description of the laboratory tests.

Except in particular situations where some knowledge of the procedure is vital for intelligent interpretation, we have not described the technical process involved in performing the laboratory tests, assuming that quality control is duly exercised by responsible institutions and laboratories.

We are grateful to Dr. Ara G. Tilkian, who wrote the chapter on diagnostic tests in cardiovascular disease. He was asked to contribute to this work because of his knowledge in this field and his current activity in the Cardiovascular Division of Stanford University Medical Center.

We would also like to express our appreciation to Mary Jo Lyon, who helped with the secretarial work in the preparation of the final manuscript, to Catherine Parker Anthony and Dr. and Mrs. Byron Schottelius, for their kind permission to use the anatomical illustrations from their books, and to Rene Fontan, for his work on the remainder of the drawings.

We are grateful to the W. B. Saunders Company and to the editors of Todd-Sanford *Clinical Diagnosis by Laboratory Methods*, and to the Lea & Febiger Company and Dr. H. Feigenbaum, author of the book *Echocardiography*, for their kind permission to reproduce the tables of normal values from their books.

The junior author would like to thank Mrs. Florence Foster, R.N., for her assistance and encouragement over the years and Mr. George P. Fee for his valuable suggestions.

Sarko M. Tilkian
Mary H. Conover

Contents

2 *Routine hematology screening, 24*

3 *Urinalysis, 35*

Appendix to Unit One

UNIT TWO

Evaluative and diagnostic laboratory tests for specific diseases

6   Diagnostic tests for renal disorders, 107

7   Diagnostic tests for gastrointestinal disorders, 120

8 *Diagnostic tests for endocrine disorders, 141*

9   *Diagnostic tests for hematologic disorders, 159*

10   *Diagnostic tests for neurologic disorders, 168*

11   *Serodiagnostic tests, 177*

Appendices

References, 212

Routine multisystem screening tests

An increase in the number, availability, and sophistication of laboratory tests has made them valuable tools in the study of clinical problems. In recent years multiphasic screening tests have been adopted widely to supplement the conventional history and physical examination. They are based on the fact that a group of laboratory determinations can now be carried out on a single specimen at a relatively low cost.

These helpful diagnostic procedures, however, do not release one from the careful study and observation of the patient, nor should they be ordered without an understanding and appreciation of their merits and limitations as well as their hazards and expense. When performed as part of the total physical examination they have the following advantages:

1. Biochemical aberrations that are usually undetectable by routine history and physical can be discovered more easily.
2. When the patient has a known disease, the screening panels serve as a gauge of the overall biochemical state relative to the existing malady.
3. When there is a diagnostic problem, the findings of the screening panels may help with the differential diagnosis.
4. They supply data concerning the biochemical parameters necessary for the safe administration of medications.

The most commonly used biochemical screening panels are routine blood chemistry, hematology, and urinalysis.

Blood chemistry usually includes calcium, phosphorus, glucose, uric acid, cholesterol, total protein, albumin, alkaline phosphatase, bilirubin, lactic dehydrogenase (LDH), serum glutamic oxalacetic transaminase (SGOT), blood urea nitrogen (BUN), creatinine, and electrolytes.

Hematology consists of a white blood count and differential, red blood count, hematocrit, hemoglobin, mean corpuscular volume, mean corpuscular hemaglobin concentration, and sedimentation rate.

The urinalysis consists of determining the pH, specific gravity, glucose, blood, protein, and a microscopic examination.

1

Blood chemistry and electrolytes

If an automated analyzer is used, a single specimen of blood may be used to determine levels of electrolytes and chemical constituents. The following tests are listed in the order which they usually appear on the automated report.

CALCIUM (Ca)

Over 98% of the calcium in the body is in the skeleton and teeth. Although the calcium in the extracellular fluid is only a small fraction of the total, its level and the level of phosphorus are regulated precisely by the parathyroid gland and the total serum protein, rarely varying more than 5% above or below normal.

Of the total plasma calcium, 50% is ionized, while most of the rest is protein bound. The ionized calcium is important in blood coagulation, in the function of the heart, muscles, and nerves, and in membrane permeability.

The parathyroid hormone raises the plasma ionized calcium concentration by acting directly on osteoclasts to release bone salts into the extracellular fluid, thus affecting both calcium and phosphate levels in the plasma. The parathyroid hormone also increases the rate of absorption of calcium from the intestines and acts on the renal tubular cells, causing calcium to be saved and phosphorus to be lost.

Two other factors important in calcium metabolism are vitamin D and the potent hypocalcemic hormone, calcitonin. Vitamin D increases the efficiency of intestinal calcium absorption, and calcitonin has opposite effects of the parathyroid hormone in that it increases renal calcium clearance.

NORMAL SERUM CALCIUM

Ionized: 4.2-5.2 mg/dl
2.1-2.6 mEq/L or 50% to 58% of total
Total: 9.0-10.6 mg/dl
4.5-5.3 mEq/L
Infants: 11-13 mg/dl

Most frequently a normal serum calcium value along with a normal overall bio-

3

chemical screening panel rules out any significant disease entity involving calcium metabolism. However, a normal calcium value may reflect significant disease in the presence of an abnormal level of phosphorus. In serum, the product of Ca × P (mg/100 ml) is normally about 50 in children. This product may be below 30 in rickets.

A normal blood calcium level in association with an elevated blood urea nitrogen (BUN) would be very suggestive of one of two things: (1) secondary hyperparathyroidism, in which case the uremia and acidosis have initially lowered the serum calcium, which in turn will stimulate the parathyroid, resulting in a normal serum calcium or (2) primary hyperparathyroidism, which would initially elevate the serum calcium. The development of secondary kidney disease and uremia would then lower the elevated calcium to normal by phosphate retention.

A normal serum calcium associated with a marked decrease in serum albumin should be considered abnormal hypercalcemia. Since about 50% of the total serum calcium is protein bound, the blood level of calcium should be depressed in the presence of hypoproteinemia. Since free calcium ions are not measured directly, the concentration of serum proteins is an important factor in estimating the level of ionized calcium in the blood.

Hypercalcemia

If all other biochemical values are normal an elevation of calcium should raise the possibility of laboratory error, and a second determination of calcium and phosphorus should then be made.

Hypercalcemia associated with hypophosphatemia is characteristic of hyperparathyroidism.

Hypercalcemia associated with hypergammaglobulinemia indicates three main possibilities: (1) sarcoidosis, (2) multiple myeloma, or (3) malignancies.

Hypercalcemia associated with metabolic alkalosis should raise the possibility of milk-alkali syndrome, particularly if there is a history of peptic ulcer, in which case there may have been ingestion of large amounts of calcium (milk) and absorbable antacids.

Hypercalcemia with a significant elevation of alkaline phosphatase may suggest Paget's disease of bone.

Other causes of hypercalcemia are severe thyrotoxicosis, malignant tumors with or without bone metastasis, and bone fractures, especially during bedrest. Hypercalcemia may also be found in idiopathic hypercalcemia, acute bone atrophy, hypervitaminosis D, polycythemia vera, some cases of acromegaly, and Cushing's syndrome with osteoporosis.

Hypocalcemia

Whenever hypocalcemia is encountered, it is advisable to perform a serum protein electrophoresis. If there is significant diminution of the albumin fraction, the hypocalcemia may not reflect true hypocalcemia and may not be significant in terms of calcium metabolism. This is termed pseudohypocalcemia. In such a situation, a reduction of albumin would also cause the serum calcium to be low.

The causes of hypocalcemia, after ruling out pseudohypocalcemia, are:

1. Hypoparathyroidism, especially if the patient has undergone thyroid or parathyroid surgery
2. Osteomalacia in adults and rickets in children due to vitamin D deficiency
3. Chronic steatorrhea, due to pancreatic insufficiency, sprue, celiac disease, or biliary obstruction, all of which cause decreased absorption of calcium from the gastrointestinal tract (malabsorption syndrome); in this case as well as in acute pancreatitis, fatty acids form calcium soaps, which precipitate, causing calcium to be lost in the feces
4. Pregnancy
5. Diuretic intake if there is a history of such intake
6. Respiratory alkalosis and hyperventilation; since alkalosis causes calcium ions to bind to protein, there is a decrease in the ionized calcium fraction
7. In newborns
8. Hypomagnesemia

Effect of calcium on the electrocardiogram

The S-T segment changes of the ECG may be very helpful in case of doubt as to laboratory error or in situations where a quick evaluation of the serum calcium level is desirable, particularly in the hyperventilation syndrome. Usually hypocalcemia causes significant prolongation of the S-T segment of the Q-T interval. Hypercalcemia causes shortening of the Q-T interval and perhaps a widening and rounding of the T waves.

PHOSPHORUS (PO₄)

The phosphorus level is usually determined in the phosphate form. It is always correlated with the calcium level. The optimal ratio is 1:1, with adequate vitamin D intake. Calcium and phosphorus determinations are always ordered together because of their close relationship. As mentioned in the discussion of calcium, the parathyroid hormone causes an increased rate of absorption of calcium and phosphorus, and causes phosphate to be lost and calcium saved as a result of its effect on renal tubular reabsorption. Phosphate is a threshold substance, and as such its loss in the urine is dependent upon both its level in the serum and the level of calcium, since if either element is in excess the other will be excreted.

Of the total phosphorus, 85% is combined with calcium in the skeleton. It is found abundantly in all tissues and is involved in almost all metabolic processes.

With these principles in mind, it is evident that, in the absence of significant glomerular disease (with normal BUN and normal creatinine), phosphate abnormalities should direct attention toward some kind of abnormality associated with the endocrine system or bone metabolism.

NORMAL SERUM PHOSPHORUS

    Adults: 1.8-2.6 mEq/L
            3.0-4.5 mg/dl
  Children: 2.3-4.1 mEq/L
            4.0-7.0 mg/dl

Hyperphosphatemia

Probably the most common cause of elevated phosphate is chronic glomerular disease with elevated BUN and creatinine. However, the importance of measuring blood phosphate and calcium levels lies in its value in diagnosing hypoparathyroidism, the hallmark of which is hyperphosphatemia in association with hypocalcemia and normal renal function.

The phosphate level may be normal or increased in both milk-alkali syndrome and sarcoidosis when normal renal function is associated with primary abnormal calcium metabolism. In the former there will be a history of peptic ulcer disease; the latter may be suggested by the Kveim test, described on p. 101 and by hyperglobulinemia and the clinical picture.

Other endocrine conditions associated with elevated phosphates include hyperthyroidism and increased growth hormone secretion. Other causes may be pseudohypoparathyroidism, fractures in the healing stage, malignant hyperpyrexia (following anesthesia), feeding newborns on unadapted cow's milk, which has a much higher phosphate content than human milk, and hypervitaminosis D.

Hypophosphatemia

Hypophosphatemia may be the result of one of the following:
1. Hyperparathyroidism, the hallmark of which is hypophosphatemia in association with hypercalcemia. Although possibly not the most common cause of decreased phosphate, this combination in the absence of significant renal disease is clinically characteristic of hyperparathyroidism.
2. Childhood rickets or adult osteomalacia, particularly if there is elevation of the alkaline phosphatase. In either of these conditions, the serum calcium may be low or normal.
3. Certain types of renal tubular acidosis, which is relatively rare and may be a single defect of phosphate reabsorption from the distal tubules (that is, phosphate diabetes) or multiple defects (De Fanconi syndrome and the aminoacidurias). These diseases may be associated with other abnormalities of amino acid metabolism, distal tubular acidosis, and acid-base abnormalities.
4. In the absence of the above conditions, hypophosphatemia may be an indication of such conditions as malabsorption syndromes and hyperinsulinism.

BLOOD GLUCOSE (Gluc)

Most carbohydrates in the diet are digested to form glucose or fructose and are taken by the portal vein to the liver, where fructose is converted to glucose. The utilization of glucose by the body cells is intimately related to insulin, the hormone secreted from the islets of Langerhans in the pancreas.

Assuming that the patient was in a fasting state when the blood for the analysis was drawn, one usually sees the following order of frequency and range for blood glucose:

1. Normal, between 80 and 100 mg/100 ml
2. Mild elevation, between 120 and 130 mg/100 ml
3. Moderate elevation, between 300 and 500 mg/100 ml
4. Marked elevation, greater than 500 mg/100 ml, associated with ketoacidosis, which is reflected by decreased CO_2 combining power
5. Marked elevation with hyperosmolar state, without ketoacidosis
6. Below the normal accepted ranges

The normal range for fasting blood sugar varies among laboratories and with the type of procedure used. One should consult the particular laboratory as to the normal range and the method used.

Since the implications of each of the above classifications are different, consideration of the blood sugar determination in these categories is advantageous.

NORMAL BLOOD GLUCOSE

Serum or plasma: 70-110 mg/100 ml
Whole blood: 60-100 mg/100 ml

Although the most commonly encountered category is a fasting blood glucose that is within normal limits, it should be remembered that a normal value rules out any significant diabetic problem, but that it does not rule out diabetes as such. Patients who have latent diabetes or prediabetes will have normal fasting blood sugars even though they are, by definition, diabetic. This is certain if both parents are known to be diabetic, if an identical twin is a known diabetic, or if the patient has diabetic vascular changes without an elevated blood sugar.

Hyperglycemia

Hyperglycemia is usually equated with diabetes. In most cases any degree of elevated blood sugar does indicate diabetes, whether the elevation is transient or permanent. However, in always equating hyperglycemia with diabetes, one runs the risk of forgetting other diseases that may be associated with hyperglycemia. For example, hyperglycemia is present in Cushing's disease or in patients being treated with steroids. It is uncertain whether the hyperglycemia in the latter situation is latent diabetes manifested as a clinical diabetes by excess steroids, or whether this kind of an elevated blood sugar is an altogether different pathophysiological entity from the well-known inherited form of diabetes mellitus. The uncertainty is compounded by the fact that one of the tests employed in the diagnosis of latent diabetes is the steroid stimulation test.

It is probably best to simply define diabetes mellitus as the hereditary disease associated with fasting hyperglycemia and found in the majority of hypergly-cemic patients. However, it bears repeating that hyperglycemia may not neces-sarily mean diabetes. A reasonably diligent search for other possible causes of hyperglycemia may produce the correct diagnosis. A glucose tolerance test is indi-cated when blood glucose levels are borderline or there is clinical evidence of hereditary diabetes.

Mild hyperglycemia (120-130 mg/100 ml)

Entities (other than diabetes) associated with mild hyperglycemia are:
1. Conditions causing elevation of blood catecholamines and steroids. The most frequent cause of this is acute stress (acute infection, myocardial infarction, and the like) which may herald the onset of hereditary diabetes.
2. Pheochromocytoma, a tumor producing adrenalin and noradrenalin.
3. Cushing's syndrome and Cushing's disease, both of which cause hyperglycemia because of elevated glucocorticoids. In Cushing's syndrome, which may be due to a pituitary adenoma, growth hormones may be involved, which definitely elevate the blood sugar.
4. Hyperthyroidism, which is suggested when mild hyperglycemia is associated with hypocholesterolemia. The increase in blood sugar is probably mediated through an increase in catecholamines.
5. Adenoma of the pancreas, producing only glucagon that antagonizes insulin, causing hyperglycemia.
6. Diuretics, mainly the thiazide diuretics. It is uncertain whether the hypergly-cemia is induced by a direct diuretic action on the pancreas or by hypokalemia, which is known to suppress the release of insulin.
7. Acute or chronic pancreatic insufficiency, the mechanism of which may be the destruction of islet cells.

Moderate hyperglycemia (300-500 mg/100 ml)

A moderate elevation in blood sugar usually leaves no doubt as to the diagnosis of diabetes mellitus. Depending on the age of the patient and other findings, a mod-erate hyperglycemia usually becomes a management problem.

Marked hyperglycemia (>500 mg/100 ml)

When a marked elevation in blood sugar is encountered, attention should im-mediately be directed to the CO_2 combining power. This is extremely important, because if the CO_2 combining power is low, the patient has uncontrolled diabetes associated with ketoacidosis, a potentially dangerous situation.

The second possibility, which is relatively rare, is a marked hyperglycemia with-out ketoacidosis (reflected by a normal CO_2 combining power). This entity, also serious, is called nonketotic and nonacidotic hyperglycemia; it is not necessarily associated with diabetes. The patient is usually very ill, with significant abnormal intermediary carbohydrate metabolism, caused by the uncoupling of oxidative phosphorylation. It is usually found in elderly patients with advanced vascular disease and anoxemia. There is associated dehydration with hypernatremia.

Hypoglycemia

The finding of a fasting hypoglycemia is quite unusual. However, once it is encountered the following conditions should be considered:

1. Pancreatic islet cell tumor, which independently secretes insulin without the associated check and balance of a normal metabolism
2. Large tumors of nonpancreatic origin, particularly large retroperitoneal sarcomas or large hepatomas.
3. Pituitary hypofunction
4. Adrenocortical hypofunction (Addison's disease); if this is the cause the patient will also have slight hyperkalemia and hyponatremia and a slightly elevated BUN
5. Acquired extensive liver disease

Other relatively rare conditions associated with hypoglycemia include glycogen storage disease; postnatal hypoglycemia in infants of diabetic mothers; and alcoholic hypoglycemia, which is usually associated with a substantial alcohol ingestion after a period of fasting.

Rarer still is hypoglycemia caused by certain amino acids (leucine hypoglycemia). One should also be aware of patients who are taking oral hypoglycemics or insulin and who may have a fasting hypoglycemia in the morning.

Reactive hypoglycemia

In functional reactive hypoglycemia, a rising blood sugar level stimulates excessive insulin secretion. In this syndrome the insulin continues to act after most of the carbohydrate has been stored or metabolized, and hypoglycemia results. A 5-hour glucose tolerance test usually detects a lowering of the blood sugar between three and five hours. Preferably, samples should be drawn every half hour.

URIC ACID

Uric acid is the end product of purine metabolism and is cleared from the plasma by glomerular filtration and perhaps by tubular secretion. One very rarely encounters a uric acid level significantly below expressed ranges. Therefore, we will not consider hypouricemia except to state that in very rare conditions, such as Wilson's disease or Fanconi syndrome, the uric acid level may be low.

NORMAL SERUM URIC ACID

Male: 2.1-7.8 mg/dl
Female: 2.0-6.4 mg/dl

In most instances a normal uric acid value is given no further attention. However, a normal uric acid level does not rule out gout, although it makes such a diagnosis unlikely.

Hyperuricemia

Hyperuricemia is usually equated with gout, in which there is a clinical picture of either tophi or acute arthritis with significant hyperuricemia.

However, mild hyperuricemia is most commonly idiopathic, in which case the patient is asymptomatic. It would be an unfortunate mistake to label every hyperuricemia "gout" and treat the hyperuricemia rather than the patient. Usually the blood uric acid reflects the balance of uric acid production and excretion.

The association of idiopathic hyperuricemia with hyperlipidemia and coronary artery disease is of clinical importance, although the reason for the association is unclear.

Another common cause of hyperuricemia is chronic renal failure. This can be ascertained relatively quickly by correlating the uric acid elevation with the creatinine and BUN, both of which will be elevated.

A differential diagnosis is necessary between hyperuricemia caused by chronic renal failure and that due to gouty nephropathy with secondary chronic renal failure. In the latter condition, which is relatively rare, it would be impossible to determine through laboratory tests which came first, the gouty nephropathy or the renal failure. In this situation the clinical picture is extremely helpful.

Other causes of hyperuricemia are congestive heart failure with decreased creatinine clearance, starvation (particularly absolute starvation of obese persons for weight reduction purposes), and certain glycogen storage diseases (Von Gierke's disease or Lesch-Nyhan syndrome).

Most of the conditions associated with the excessive production of uric acid belong to the lympho- and myeloproliferative diseases, such as acute or chronic leukemia, both leukocytic and granulocytic, multiple myeloma, or any other malignancy associated with rapid destruction of nucleic acid and purine products. Chemotherapy or radiotherapy in these disorders may further elevate the uric acid level.

Several drugs are associated with hyperuricemia. The most common of these are the diuretics, particularly the thiazide diuretics, which impair uric acid clearance by the kidneys.

In addition, hyperuricemia may be found in Tangier disease (alpha lipoprotein deficiency), hypoparathyroidism, primary hyperoxaluria, lead poisoning due to moonshine whiskey (saturnine gout), and excessive ethyl alcohol intake.

CHOLESTEROL (Chol)

Cholesterol exists in the body in both a free and an esterified form (combined with a fatty acid). Most of the ingested cholesterol is esterified in the intestine and absorbed as such into the lymph. The liver synthesizes cholesterol from acetate. This synthesis is presumably inhibited by a high level of circulating cholesterol.

Cholesterol is used in the body to form cholic acid in the liver, which in turn forms bile salts, important for fat digestion. A small quantity of cholesterol is used in the formation of hormones by the adrenal glands, ovaries, and testes. A large amount is used to make the skin highly resistant to the absorption of water-soluble substances.

The concentration of cholesterol in the blood is influenced by thyroid hormones and estrogens, both of which cause a decrease. Plasma cholesterol is elevated when biliary flow is obstructed, and also in hereditary hypercholesterolemia and untreated diabetes mellitus, in spite of a decrease in cholesterol synthesis in diabetes.

There is popular interest in cholesterol values since hypercholesterolemia is a much publicized risk factor for coronary artery disease. This is discussed in Chapter 4. It is important to keep in mind that normal values for cholesterol are arbitrarily defined and show much variation in different populations and age groups.

NORMAL SERUM CHOLESTEROL

150-250 mg/dl (varies with diet and age, and from country to country)

Marked hypercholesterolemia (>400 mg/dl)

Marked hypercholesterolemia is seen in:
1. Liver disease associated with biliary obstruction; in this condition elevated alkaline phosphatase and bilirubin levels accompany hypercholesterolemia
2. Nephrotic stage of glomerulonephritis; elevated BUN and creatinine may be present
3. Familial hypercholesterolemia, a genetically transmitted disorder, more pronounced if homozygous

Other causes of hypercholesterolemia are hypothyroidism, pancreatectomy, and pancreatic dysfunction such as that in diabetes mellitus and chronic pancreatitis.

Significant hypocholesterolemia (<150 mg/dl)

A significantly low blood cholesterol may reflect dietary habits, malnutrition, extensive liver disease, and possibly hyperthyroidism, which does produce a low normal serum cholesterol.

In liver disease it is advisable to fractionate the cholesterol to the esterified form, since esterification is affected by liver damage much more than is the total cholesterol.

Other conditions that may be associated with hypcholesterolemia are severe sepsis, anemia (megaloblastic and hypochromic), serum α and β lipoprotein deficiency, and certain enzyme deficiencies associated with cholesterol metabolism.

TOTAL PROTEIN AND ALBUMIN/GLOBULIN RATIO
(tot prot and A/G ratio)

Plasma proteins serve as a source of rapid replacement of tissue proteins during tissue depletion, as buffers in acid-base balance, and as transporters of constituents of the blood, such as lipids, vitamins, hormones, iron, copper, and certain enzymes. The antibodies of the body are contained in the gamma globulins and a number of the plasma proteins participate in blood coagulation. Of the total protein, between 52% and 68% is albumin. This fraction is responsible for about 80% of the colloid oncotic pressure in the serum. The capillary walls are impermeable to the proteins in plasma. The proteins, therefore, exert an osmotic force across the capillary wall (oncotic pressure) that tends to pull water into the blood.

Although the total protein and A/G ratio is still a commonly employed test, it is gradually being replaced by serum protein electrophoresis, which more clearly delineates the different albumin and globulin fractions.

Electrophoresis is the migration of charged particles in an electrolyte solution in response to an electrical current passed through the solution. The proteins move at different rates because each is different in electrical charge, size, and shape. Thus the proteins tend to separate into distinct layers.

Immunoelectrophoresis is a combination of electrophoresis and immunodiffusion to permit analysis of the various immunoglobulin fractions.

NORMAL TOTAL PROTEIN AND ALBUMIN/GLOBULIN RATIO

Total: 6.0-7.8 gm/dl
Albumin: 3.2-4.5 gm/dl
Globulin: 2.3-3.5 gm/dl

Hypoalbuminemia

A depressed albumin with a slightly elevated globulin is a reversal of the A/G ratio and suggests chronic liver disease. Thus, an albumin of 2.5 gm and below, with a globulin of 3 gm/100 ml and a total protein in the range of 5.5 gm/100 ml is extremely suggestive of chronic liver disease.

Other conditions associated with hypoalbuminemia are significant malnutrition (especially protein), nephrotic syndrome, and malabsorption syndromes, particularly protein-losing enteropathies.

Normal total protein, low albumin, and elevated globulin

When a normal total protein is associated with a low normal albumin and an elevated globulin the A/G ratio is reversed. This type of laboratory picture is suggestive of diseases with hypergammaglobulinemia and includes the myeloproliferative diseases such as multiple myeloma, Hodgkin's disease, and leukemias; the chronic granulomatous infectious diseases such as tuberculosis, brucellosis, collagen disease, chronic active hepatitis, and sarcoidosis.

Under the above cirumstances one is obliged to use serum protein electrophoresis to determine if one is dealing with a broad band of gamma globulin or a sharp peak in the gamma, alpha I, alpha II, or beta range. The latter would be indicative of variants of multiple myeloma and macroglobulinemias.

THE ENZYMES

A usual analysis includes the following enzymes: alkaline phosphatase (alk phos), lactic dehydrogenase (LDH), and serum glutamic-oxaloacetic transaminase (SGOT).

Enzymes are found in all tissues. They are complex, naturally occurring compounds that catalyze the biochemical reactions of the body; that is, they speed up reactions that might otherwise proceed very slowly. Each tissue has its own specific enzyme, with one enzyme being common to more than one type of tissue. For example, alkaline phosphatase is found mainly in bone and liver and in small amounts in kidneys and the gastrointestinal tract. SGOT is found mainly in heart and skeletal muscle and in the liver, kidneys, and red blood cells.

One looks for elevation of these enzymes in the laboratory examination, the implication being that the particular tissue is damaged enough to release significant quantities of the enzyme into the blood.

Alkaline phosphatase (alk phos)

Alkaline phosphatase is an enzyme that mediates some of the complex reactions of bone formation. When the osteoblasts are actively depositing bone matrix, they secrete large quantities of alkaline phosphatase.

The two main sources of alkaline phosphatase are bone and liver. Consequently, an elevation of alkaline phosphatase immediately directs attention to either liver problems or bone disease which will correlate with clinical findings, such as jaundice indicating liver disease. The chemical composition of the enzyme from each of these sources is slightly different, so that if the enzyme is fractionated one of the fractions (isoenzymes) is specific to the particular organ or tissue from which it came. For clinical purposes, the isoenzymes are not separated, although in highly specialized laboratories the different isoenzymes can be isolated by the process of electrophoresis (p. 12).

NORMAL ALKALINE PHOSPHATASE (TOTAL SERUM)

Adults: 1.5-4.5 U/dl (Bodansky)
        4-13 U/dl (King-Armstrong)
        0.8-2.3 U/ml (Bessey-Lowry)
        15-35 U/ml (Shinowara-Jones-Reinhart)
Children: 5.0-14.0 U/dl (Bodansky)
        3.4-9.0 U/ml (Bessey-Lowry)
        15-30 U/dl (King-Armstrong)

Extreme elevation of alkaline phosphatase with liver disease

When an extremely high level of alkaline phosphatase (15 U/dl or more, Bodansky) is associated with liver disease (abnormal liver function tests) the following are indicated:
1. Early phases of obstructive jaundice, with obstruction at the level of the major biliary ducts (gallstone or carcinoma of the head of the pancreas). In this case the patient initially has a slight bilirubinemia; it gradually increases and is accompanied by the extremely high alkaline phosphatase.
2. Space-occupying lesions of the liver, either widespread metastatic liver disease or an obstructive tumor of the biliary ducts. The alkaline phosphatase in the latter case is presumed to come from the cells lining the bile ducts. The obstruction and the damage cause the enzyme to leak from the cells and appear in the bloodstream.

Extreme elevation of alkaline phosphatase without liver disease

In the absence of any indication of liver disease (normal liver function tests), extreme elevation of alkaline phosphatase along with some indication of bone pathology suggests Paget's disease of bone, in which the highest level of this enzyme is found, especially if osteogenic sarcoma develops.

Extreme elevations of alkaline phosphatase can also be found in carcinomas metastatic to bone.

Moderate and slight elevation of alkaline phosphatase with liver disease

In the presence of liver disease, moderate elevation (8-12 U/dl Bodansky) of alkaline phosphatase is usually associated with cholangiolitic hepatitis.

A slight elevation of alkaline phosphatase in the presence of liver disease usually indicates cirrhosis of the liver with some active hepatitis.

Moderate and slight elevation of alkaline phosphatase without liver disease

In the absence of liver involvement (normal liver function tests) and in the presence of hypercalcemia an elevated alkaline phosphatase level indicates the possibility of hyperparathyroidism. In this situation there is a slight elevation of the enzyme in the initial stage. At a later stage there may be significant elevations. In secondary and tertiary hyperparathyroidism, borderline elevations may be encountered.

If other indicators of bone pathology (bone scan revealing evidence of bone disease) are present, mild to moderate elevations of alkaline phosphatase can be seen in osteomalacia. Usually such elevation will supply the differential diagnosis between osteomalacia and osteoporosis. In the latter condition the alkaline phosphatase is normal.

A slight elevation of alkaline phosphatase also occurs in childhood and during the growth period, in pregnancy, and in rickets.

Low alkaline phosphatase

A low alkaline phosphatase level is usually not of much clinical significance. However, if a low value of this enzyme persists, one should consider some of the extremely rare entities such as hypophosphatasia, achondroplasia, cretinism, and vitamin C deficiency.

Lactic dehydrogenase (LDH)

Lactic dehydrogenase is an enzyme that catalyzes the reversible oxidation of lactic acid to pyruvic acid. It is present in nearly all metabolizing cells, with highest concentrations in heart, liver, kidney, brain, skeletal muscle, and erythrocytes. Damage to nearly any tissue can cause this enzyme to be released into the blood stream. The origin of the release cannot be determined by routine examination. However, recently LDH has been separated into five isoenzymes, thus sharpening its diagnostic value. Electrophoresis is used to separate the isoenzymes of LDH, thus determining the source of an elevation of this enzyme.

One should be aware of the possibility of falsely elevated LDH levels because of hemolyzed blood specimens. Thus, when all other parameters are normal except the LDH, the test should be repeated before any further investigations are undertaken.

NORMAL LDH (SERUM)

   80-120 Wacker units
   71-207 IU/L
   150-450 Wroblewski units

Extreme elevation of LDH (>1500 Wroblewski units)

The highest values of this enzyme are seen in patients with myocardial infarction, hemolytic disorders, and pernicious anemia.

Slight elevation of LDH (500-700 Wroblewski units)

Slight elevations that are persistent should direct attention to the following disease entities: chronic viral hepatitis; malignancies of skeletal muscle, liver, kidney, brain, blood, and heart; destruction of pulmonary tissue (pneumonia and pulmonary emboli); generalized viral infection involving multiple organs (infectious mononucleosis); low grade hemolytic disorders; cerebrovascular accidents with brain damage; and renal tissue destruction (renal infarcts, infections, or malignancies).

Serum glutamic-oxaloacetic transaminase (SGOT)

The transaminase enzymes catalyze the conversion of one amino acid to the corresponding keto acid with simultaneous conversion of another keto acid to an amino acid. Transamination reactions occur in many tissues.

SGOT is found mainly in heart muscle and the liver and to a certain degree in skeletal muscle, kidney, and red blood cells. Normally almost all of this enzyme is intracellular. Following injury or death of physiologically active cells, the enzyme is released into the circulation. Elevated values may be found eight hours after injury and should peak in twenty-four to thirty-six hours if the original episode is not repeated. It usually falls to normal in four to six days. The amount of SGOT in the blood is in direct proportion to the number of cells damaged and the interval of time between tissue injury and the test.

NORMAL SGOT (SERUM)

   8-33 U/ml

Extreme elevation of SGOT (>1000 U/ml)

There are extremely high levels of this enzyme in the acute stages of severe fulminating hepatitis in which there is massive destruction of liver tissue, in severe liver necrosis, and in skeletal muscle damage.

Following the acute stage in hepatocellular damage, the highest values of SGOT are found in acute myocardial infarction, depending on the size of the infarct and the time relationship between the onset of the infarct and the drawing of the blood.

Minor elevation of SGOT (40-100 U/ml)

Minor elevations of SGOT can be seen in congestive heart failure, tachyarrhythmias in the presence of shock, pericarditis, pulmonary infarction, and dissecting aneurysm, as well as in cirrhosis, cholangiolitic jaundice, metastatic liver disease, skeletal muscle disease, posttraumatic states, and generalized infections such as infectious mononucleosis.

BILIRUBIN (total serum)

Bilirubin is formed from the hemoglobin of destroyed erythrocytes by the reticuloendothelial system and is the predominant pigment of the bile. Being a by-product of hemoglobin metabolism, it is a waste product and thus must be excreted.

Bilirubin exists in two forms in the body, soluble (conjugated or "direct-reacting") and protein bound (unconjugated or "indirect-reacting"). The routine examination does not differentiate between the two, and further tests are run if the total bilirubin level is elevated. These tests and normal bilirubin physiology are discussed in Chapter 7 on pp. 135-137.

NORMAL BILIRUBIN (SERUM)

Total: 0.1-1.2 mg/dl
Newborn total: 1-12 mg/dl

A normal level of total bilirubin rules out any significant impairment of the excretory function of the liver or hemolysis.

Greatly elevated total bilirubin (>12 mg/dl)

A markedly elevated total bilirubin level along with a significant drop in hemoglobin and significant reticulocytosis is highly indicative of the possibility of massive hemolysis. Further tests show the bilirubin to be of the indirect-reacting type (Chapter 7, pp. 135 and 136).

If the majority of the greatly elevated bilirubin level is of the direct-reacting type (Chapter 7, pp. 135 and 136) the indication is that of obstructive jaundice in the form of obstructive phase of hepatitis, cholangiolitis, and lower biliary tree obstruction by either calculus or carcinoma.

BLOOD UREA NITROGEN (BUN)

Urea, formed in the liver by the deamination of amino acids, is the primary method of nitrogen excretion. Urea, then, is the end product of protein metabolism and is formed in the liver. After synthesis, urea travels through the blood and is excreted in the urine.

NORMAL BUN

8-18 mg/dl

Elevated BUN

Acute or chronic renal failure is the most common cause of high BUN levels. In prerenal failure, a low renal blood supply, such as occurs with congestive heart failure, leads to reduced glomerular filtration and therefore an elevated BUN. In renal failure, damage to the nephrons, such as occurs with nephritis or pyelonephritis, leads to faulty urine formation and excretion. As a result, the blood urea nitrogen begins to rise when the glomerular filtration rate falls below 50 ml/min (the normal in an average-size man is approximately 125 ml/min).

Postrenal failure due to urinary tract obstructions can also cause uremia. Prostatic enlargement is probably the most common cause of urinary tract obstruction.

Other causes of borderline elevated levels of BUN are unusually high protein intake and excessive body protein catabolism such as occurs with sepsis or fever and gastrointestinal bleeding.

SERUM CREATININE (Creat)

Creatinine is a waste product of creatine, which is present in skeletal muscle as creatine phosphate, a high energy compound.

Serum creatinine determination is another test of renal function, reflecting the balance between its production (proportional to the body's muscle mass), and filtration by the renal glomerulus.

NORMAL CREATININE (SERUM)

0.6-1.2 mg/dl

Elevated serum creatinine

Serum creatinine is elevated in all diseases of the kidney where 50% or more of the nephrons are destroyed.

Nonrenal causes of elevation or fluctuation in serum creatinine levels are few, making this a more specific test of renal failure. People with large muscle mass or patients with acromegaly may have values slightly over the normal range in the presence of normal kidney function.

ELECTROLYTES

The serum electrolyte analysis includes sodium (Na), potassium (K), chloride (Cl), and CO_2 combining power. The levels of these electrolytes in the blood are the outcome of fine regulatory mechanisms of ionic charges and the osmotic balance of the extracellular fluid. This is accomplished by the marvelous adaptation of the kidneys, lungs, and endocrine system to varying and multidirectional forces. The kidneys and the lungs are involved in electrical balance, while osmotic balance is finely governed by the endocrine system, with the hypothalamus, posterior pituitary gland, and kidneys being intricately interrelated.

It is apparent, then, that the determination of the serum level of a single electrolyte is insufficient for an overall evaluation of the patient's metabolic state. When one wishes to determine the serum level of any electrolyte, the whole series should be ordered. This approach will have a profound bearing on the correct interpretation and evaluation of the patient's electrolyte status.

The following example is given to emphasize the importance of a complete electrolyte analysis. A serum potassium level of 4.5 mEq/L means one thing if the CO_2 combining power is 35 mEq/L and means something altogether different if the CO_2

combining power is 10 mEq/L. In the first case, the patient probably has a metabolic alkalosis. This would cause the potassium to migrate into the cell and be excreted in the urine. A serum potassium of 4.5 mEq/L does not, then really reflect a true hypokalemia, since when the alkalosis is corrected the potassium will return to its extracellular position.

In the second case (CO_2 combining power of 10 mEq/L), the patient probably has a metabolic acidosis. This would cause the potassium to leave the cell. A serum potassium of 4.5 mEq/L would, then, reflect a much lower potassium, since the available potassium will migrate back into the cell when the acidosis is corrected.

In addition to electrolyte determination, it is extremely important that the blood urea nitrogen (BUN) or creatinine be determined as well. This serves two purposes. First, serum electrolyte values have one implication in the presence of an elevated BUN level with the associated metabolic acidosis, whereas when the BUN level is normal the implication changes. In addition, the BUN is a relatively good indication of the patient's overall water metabolism and hydration status, which has a pronounced effect on the different electrolytes. Second, if therapy must be instituted, particularly potassium replacement, it is essential to know kidney function. Preferably a creatinine clearance is ordered. However, if this is not available, at least one BUN determination is ordered so that the patient's condition may be managed safely.

It is preferable to measure the arterial pH, P_{O_2} and P_{CO_2} directly because the pH affects and is affected by the serum electrolyte level. This is particularly true in complex metabolic and/or respiratory acid-base problems, in which it is extremely difficult to evaluate the patient's electrolytes without knowing the arterial blood gases and pH.

Serum electrolyte levels may vary from moment to moment and are, therefore, only a rough indicator of the total body concentration of the ions. For example, in the condition known as dilutional hyponatremia the serum sodium level is below normal, but the total body sodium is increased.

There is no direct way of measuring intracellular levels of electrolytes. It is known, however, that the Q-T interval and U wave of the electrocardiogram reflect the ratio of intracellular and extracellular electrolytes. Initial information about the patient's overall electrolyte and acid-base state, therefore, may be drawn from this source.

Keeping in mind the above principles and problems, one can evaluate the electrolytes much more rationally and obtain a more significant insight into the patient's overall metabolic state. At the present time electrolyte determinations are usually performed in critical care units and in hospital environments. However, the value of electrolyte determination is being appreciated more and more in the daily office practice of physicians, particularly in view of the large number of medications employed that alter electrolytes and body water metabolism.

Collecting and handling the specimen

When blood is being drawn for electrolyte determination, the procedure should be as atraumatic as possible, and the blood obtained should be centrifuged quickly.

If there is any hemolysis this fact should be noted, because tissue breakdown or hemolysis will cause a false elevation of serum potassium levels.

Serum sodium (Na)

Sodium is the major cation of the extracellular fluid, playing an important part in the regulation of acid-base equilibrium, protecting the body against excessive fluid loss, and preserving the normal function of muscle tissue.

NORMAL SERUM SODIUM

136-142 mEq/L

Hypernatremia

Hypernatremia in the normally functioning individual is very uncommon. The most frequent cause of hypernatremia is seen in the critical care unit, where excess intravenous sodium is given to an unconscious patient whose thirst mechanism is absent. Serum sodium levels have a strong influence on the body's osmoreceptors, and in the healthy individual this initiates the thirst mechanism. The individual then drinks water until the serum sodium level is back to normal.

Hyperglycemia is associated with hypernatremia in some rare hypothalamic lesions, head trauma, and hyperosmolar states. Other causes of hypernatremia are dehydration and steroid (mineralocorticoid) administration or excess.

Hyponatremia

Hyponatremia is more frequently encountered clinically than is hypernatremia. In the ambulatory patient and in those seem in the physician's office, hyponatremia may reflect or be associated with diminution of total body sodium, normal body sodium, or excess body sodium.

Hyponatremia associated with an absolute sodium loss. Hyponatremia is associated with absolute sodium loss in the following conditions:

1. Addison's disease; in the absence of adrenal steroids, sodium reabsorption is impaired and the clinical picture is that of hyponatremia, hyperkalemia, and mild dehydration, reflected by a slight BUN elevation
2. Chronic sodium-losing nephropathy; this is probably a more frequent cause than Addison's disease, and may be a stage in chronic glomerulonephritis, pyelonephritis, manifested by abnormal renal function tests and an elevated BUN
3. Loss of gastrointestinal secretions by vomiting, diarrhea, or tube drainage, with replacement of fluid but not electrolytes
4. Loss of sodium from the skin through diaphoresis or burns, with replacement of fluids but not electrolytes
5. Loss of sodium from the kidneys through the use of diuretics (mercurial, chlorothiazide) and in chronic renal insufficiency with acidosis
6. Metabolic loss of sodium through starvation with acidosis and diabetic acidosis
7. Loss of sodium from serous cavities through paracentesis or thoracentesis

Dilution hyponatremia. Excessive water, or dilutional hyponatremia, is associated with either normal or even excess total body sodium concentrations and is found in the following conditions: chronic diuretic use with sodium restriction, secondary hyperaldosteronemia, hepatic failure with ascites, congestive heart failure, excessive water administration, acute or chronic renal insufficiency (oliguria), and diabetic acidosis (therapy without adequate sodium replacement).

Hyponatremia associated with inappropriate antidiuretic hormone syndrome. In this condition the patient continues reabsorbing water from the distal tubules and excreting a concentrated urine in spite of serum hypoosmolarity. Inappropriate antidiuretic hormone syndrome has been described in association with various other diseases such as bronchogenic carcinoma (releasing ADH-like chemicals), pulmonary infections, and metabolic diseases such as porphyria.

Hyponatremia associated with intracellular potassium depletion. An impairment of the sodium-potassium pump mechanism results in an excessive intracellular sodium influx and potassium efflux. The potassium is then lost in the urine, leaving the patient with a normal serum potassium level and low serum sodium level, which reflects the quantity of intracellular sodium influx and equivalent potassium loss.

Serum potassium (K)

Potassium is the major cation of the intracellular fluid, functioning as sodium does in the extracellular fluid, by influencing acid-base balance, osmotic pressure, and cellular membrane potential.

Serum potassium levels are profoundly affected by momentary acid-base changes. A discussion of serum potassium can be divided into three major categories: the hyperkalemias, normokalemia with normal or decreased total body potassium, and hypokalemia, which is usually associated with decreased total body potassium levels.

NORMAL SERUM POTASSIUM

3.8-5.0 mEq/L

Hyperkalemia

Hyperkalemia is countered most frequently in renal failure. It is rarely developed by oral potassium chloride ingestion with normal kidneys and with normal creatinine clearance.

Addison's disease, accompanied by hypovolemia and retention of blood urea nitrogen, is the second most frequent clinical condition associated with hyperkalemia.

A relatively rare condition, called pseudohyperkalemia, is suspected when one encounters hyperkalemia without electrocardiographic evidence. Once documented, pseudohyperkalemia should suggest a myeloproliferative disease such as thrombocytosis.

Normokalemia with decreased total body potassium

The most common clinically encountered cause of normal potassium serum levels with decreased total body potassium levels is chronic diuretic use with inadequate potassium chloride supplementation. Other causes will be discussed under hypokalemia.

The following are a few clues that may be helpful in determining total body potassium depletion with normokalemia:

1. Alkalosis; this can be verified either directly or by arterial blood pH measurement or indirectly by the elevation of the CO_2 combining power in the absence of chronic obstructive lung disease.
2. In the presence of significant hypochloremia and alkalosis, significant total body potassium depletion, not reflected in the serum, may exist.
3. A cellular level aberration of Na-K dependent ATPase and the Na-K pump may cause gradual cellular potassium depletion and may be reflected by hyponatremia rather than hypokalemia.
4. The presence of a U wave on the ECG should suggest cellular potassium depletion.

Hypokalemia

Most often, significant hypokalemia reflects total body depletion of potassium, which may have profound metabolic consequences.

Causes of hypokalemia are as follows:

1. Iatrogenic causes
   a. Diuretic therapy that depletes the body of potassium and chloride
   b. Diuretic therapy with supplementation of potassium and not chloride, causing a continual alkalosis with only a partial correction of the hypokalemia
2. Endocrine causes
   a. Cushing's syndrome
   b. Primary or secondary hyperaldosteronism associated with chronic congestive heart failure
   c. Liver disease with ascites
   d. Excessive ingestion of licorice, which contains a chemical very similar to aldosterone; the symptoms are, therefore, those of primary aldosteronism
   e. Antiinflammatory drugs, indomethacin, phenylbutazone, and steroids and sex hormones, particularly estrogens
   f. Conditions associated with hyperreninemia, when an elevated renin introduced into the system can cause a secondary aldosteronemia; such conditions include malignant hypertension, hypertensive disease, and occasionally unilateral renal vascular hypertension
3. Poor dietary habits and crash diets with inadequate intake of potassium
4. Chronic stress
5. Excessive loss of potassium without adequate replacement
   a. Gastrointestinal tract (chronic diarrhea, malabsorption syndrome)
   b. Perspiration and chronic fever
6. Renal losses of potassium associated with either potassium-losing nephropathy or other kinds of renal tubular acidosis typically involving hypokalemia in association with acidosis and hypochloremia

Electrocardiographic recognition of hyperkalemia and hypokalemia

The electrocardiogram is a very sensitive indicator of the ratio of intracellular to extracellular potassium and shows signs of hypokalemia even when the serum potassium level is still within normal limits. Hypokalemia and hyperkalemia threaten cardiac safety. It is, therefore, important to know the changes that a potassium deficit or excess will initiate on the ECG. This is discussed in Chapter 4 of Unit Two.

Serum chloride (Cl)

Chloride, chiefly an extracellular ion, is present in large quantities in the serum, exerting an important influence on acid-base balance and osmotic pressure.

NORMAL SERUM CHLORIDE

95-103 mEq/L

Hyperchloremia

Hyperchloremia is most frequently associated with renal tubular acidosis, decreased CO_2 combining power, and hypokalemia.

Hypochloremia

Most often, hypochloremia is associated with hypokalemia and alkalosis and has been termed hypokalemic-chloremic alkalosis. In such a situation the electrolyte analysis reflects low potassium, low chloride, and elevated CO_2 combining power. Most of the conditions associated with hypokalemia and alkalosis are also associated with hypochloremia.

Hypochloremia may also be associated with a normal serum potassium if the patient's potassium deficiency is being corrected with potassium preparations that do not contain chloride, or if the patient is receiving potassium-saving diuretics. These facts bring into focus two points of clinical importance: (1) potassium replacement therapy should be accompanied by a one-to-one ratio of potassium to chloride and (2) when potassium-saving diuretics are used one should watch very closely for the possible development of hypochloremia and hypochloremic alkalosis.

Carbon dioxide (CO₂) combining power

The CO_2 combining power determination is the usual laboratory test done for the detection of acid-base abnormalities. Since direct determination of the pH of the blood is not clinically practical in ordinary circumstances, the CO_2 capacity or CO_2 combining power is used instead. This test measures the total carbonic acid (H_2CO_3) and bicarbonate (HCO_3) in the plasma.

NORMAL CO₂ COMBINING POWER

24-30 mM/L

Elevated CO₂ combining power

In the absence of chronic obstructive lung disease, elevated CO_2 combining power indicates serum alkalosis and intracellular acidosis, which are most frequently associated with hypokalemia and hypochloremia.

Low CO_2 combining power

A low CO_2 combining power occurs in conditions associated with metabolic acidosis such as uremic acidosis, diabetic ketoacidosis, lactic acidosis, and renal tubular acidosis. However, if the arterial blood pH is determined and found to be elevated (alkalosis), a low CO_2 combining power would indicate respiratory alkalosis as seen in the hyperventilation syndrome.

CHAPTER 2

Routine hematology screening

In a complete blood count (CBC) a routine hematology screening includes the following determinations: white blood cell count (WBC), red blood cell count (RBC), hematocrit (Hct), hemoglobin (Hgb), and differential white cell count (Diff). The differential states the neutrophils, lymphocytes, monocytes, eosinophils, basophils, and any abnormal cells as a percent of the total WBC count.

A complete hematology examination also includes the indices, which are mean cell volume (MCV), mean cell hemoglobin (MCH), and mean cell hemoglobin concentration (MCHC). In addition, a careful inspection of the peripheral blood smear is important, as is a sedimentation rate (Sed rate or ESR).

With an accurate determination of these values, approximately 70% to 80% of the hematologic diagnosis can be made, as well as a significant amount of information gathered for the purpose either of evaluating the stages of a particular disease or of diagnosing some disease entities not directly related to the hematopoietic system.

Each hematologic measurement will be discussed separately. However, it should be emphasized that since the elements of the blood are closely interrelated, absolute values can be meaningless if the whole hematologic examination is not taken into consideration. For example, a WBC count without a differential may be normal, even in the presence of severe sepsis. In this case, a differential would reveal an extreme increase in the percentage of segmented bands.

WHITE BLOOD CELL COUNT (WBC)

The white blood cell count (WBC) expresses the number of WBCs in one microliter of whole blood. The correct WBC count can be obtained by multiplying the figure obtained from the automated Coulter counter by 1000. For example, a WBC count reported to be 7.25 should be interpreted as 7250 WBCs per microliter of whole blood.

Absolute determination of the leukocytes (total white blood cells) gives only partial information. Unless an accurate differential white cell count is done, significant pathology or information can be missed, as in the case cited above.

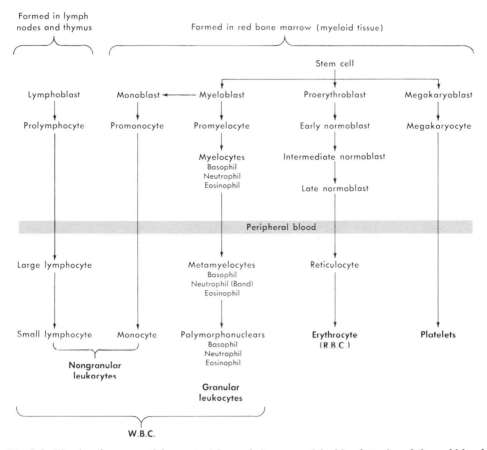

Fig. 2-1. The development of the various formed elements of the blood. In the adult, red blood cells, the granular white blood cells, monocytes, and platelets are formed in the bone marrow. The lymphocytes are formed mainly in the lymph nodes and thymus.

White blood cells (leukocytes) are either granular or nongranular. The granular leukocytes are the basophils, neutrophils, and eosinophils. The nongranular leukocytes are the lymphocytes and monocytes. (See Fig. 2-1.)

Granulocytes

Neutrophils, eosinophils, and basophils are formed from stem cells in the bone marrow. Their nuclei have two to five or more lobes, and they are therefore called polymorphonuclear. Neutrophils are so named because they stain with neutral dyes. Eosinophils stain with acid dye and basophils stain with basic dyes.

In a healthy person, the number of granulocytes is regulated at a constant level. However, when infection occurs, the number in the blood rises dramatically. When bacteria invade the body, the bone marrow is stimulated to produce and release large numbers of neutrophils, which are phagocytic. The basophils contain heparin, but their role is uncertain. Eosinophils phagocytize antigen-antibody complexes. There-fore, in patients with allergic diseases the circulating eosinophil level is often elevated.

Nongranular leukocytes

Monocytes arise in the bone marrow and migrate into inflammatory exudates, but not as rapidly as the neutrophils. Monocytosis is seen in chronic inflammatory dis-orders.

Lymphocytes are formed in the thymus, in lymph nodes, and in bone marrow. Lymphocytes derived from the thymus are longer-lived than those derived from the lymph nodes and bone marrow. The small lymphocytes are capable of producing a specific anitbody in response to an antigenic challenge.

Normal WBC count

The normal WBC count is usually between 4500 and 11,000/cu mm and may vary in a particular individual during a particular time of day. A minor variation outside the normal range is not significant as long as the differential count and the peripheral blood smear are both normal. However, some early disorder, whether infectious or myeloproliferative, is not necessarily ruled out.

Leukocytosis mild to moderate (11,000-17,000/cu mm)

Mild to moderate elevation of the WBC count usually indicates infectious disease, mainly of bacterial etiology. Usually the leukocytosis increases with the severity of the infection. However, there are exceptions to this rule, particularly in elderly patients in whom severe sepsis can coexist with only a modest leukocytosis. As mentioned pre-viously, the differential WBC count is of additional help.

Leukemoid reaction

Occasionally such massive leukocytosis accompanies a systemic disease that the blood picture of leukemia is simulated. When a blood picture looks like leukemia but is not, the term "leukemoid reaction" is used. Severe sepsis, military tuberculosis, and other nonmalignant infectious conditions are among the more common causes.

Leukopenia

A decreased absolute WBC count (leukopenia) can be mild (3000-5000/cu mm), moderate (1500-3000/cu mm), or extremely severe (<1500/cu mm), and may be asso-ciated with diminution of the WBC count as a whole, decreases in neutrophils, or diminution of all the blood particles (pancytopenia).

Leukopenia associated with neutropenia

The most common causes of a mild to moderate decrease in neutrophils are:
1. Familial benign neutropenia, usually accompanied by moderate monocytosis up to 50%
2. Acute viral infections
3. Starvation neutropenia (anorexia nervosa)

4. Primary and secondary splenic neutropenia associated with Felty's syndrome, portal hypertension, lymphoma, and some specific bacterial and protozoal infections
5. Drug-induced neutropenia, with the following drugs implicated: phenothiazines (Thorazine group), antithyroid drugs, sulfonamides, phenylbutazone, chloramphenicol, phenindione, and aminophylline, or their derivatives
6. Acute alcoholic ingestion

Leukopenia associated with eosinopenia

The most common causes of mild to moderate decrease in eosinophils are acute and chronic stress, either emotional or somatic; and endocrine causes such as excess ACTH, cortisone, or epinephrine, intermenstrual period, certain diurnal variations, and acromegaly.

Granulocytopenia

From a practical point of view, one determination of neutropenia in the absence of any other indication of disease should be regarded as benign, possibly diurnal, or maybe stress related. However, granulocytopenia associated with any other disease states should be evaluated according to the following causes:
1. Acute hypersensitive reactions
2. Steroids (ACTH, thyroxine, epinephrine, estrogen)
3. Diurnal changes
4. Hyperthyroidism
5. Pituitary basophilism
6. Radiation therapy
7. Acute and chronic infection
8. Ovulation
9. Pregnancy
10. Aging

The differential count

The differential count is performed on a peripheral blood smear for the purpose of identifying the different types of leukocytes. Red blood cell and platelet morphology can also be evaluated in this way.

Among the leukocytes, the neutrophils are usually the most abundant cells seen on the peripheral smear, comprising 56% of the total white blood cell count. Normally 2.7% will be eosinophils, 0.3% will be basophils, and 34% will be lymphocytes.

When an extremely high leukocytosis is reported, one should very carefully inspect the peripheral smear. An accurate differential count may be enough to make the diagnosis of myelocytic leukemia or lymphocytic leukemia.

A thorough examination of the peripheral blood smear should routinely include the following:
1. A diligent search should be made for abnormal lymphocytes and monocytes that

may indicate some specific disease such as infectious mononucleosis. This disease is diagnosed by the Downey cells found in the peripheral smear.

2. Look for an extreme shift to the left, which implies a significant number of early neutrophils and band forms rather than lobulations. This shift will indicate some kind of acute stress on the bone marrow or severe bacterial disease causing the release of an early granulocytic series and will, at the same time, give the interpreter some indication of the stage and severity of the disease.

3. Abnormal granulations in the leukocytes may give an index of toxicity generated by a specific disease (toxic granulation).

4. In examining the leukocytes, one may gain significant information by counting the lobulations of hypersegmented neutrophils. Hyperlobulation (from three to six) or segmentation of neutrophils is suggestive of vitamin B_{12} deficiency or folic acid deficiency.

Neutrophilic leukocytosis

The most commonly encountered conditions that manifest a mild to moderate leukocytosis of neutrophilic origin are the bacterial infections, inflammatory disorders, tumors, physical and emotional stimuli, stresses, and drugs.

The bacterial infections are usually moderately severe bacterial pneumonias or systemic infections, which are sometimes coccal.

The inflammatory but noninfectious diseases causing neutrophilic leukocytosis are rheumatic fever, collagen disease, rheumatoid arthritis, vasculitis, pancreatitis, thyroiditis, and tumors and carcinomas, particularly gastric, bronchogenic, uterine, pancreatic, squamous cell, lymphatic, and those of Hodgkin's disease. Additional conditions are burns, crush injury, infarctions, and poisoning with carbon monoxide or lead.

Stresses that produce neutrophilic leukocytosis can be extreme cold, heat, exercise, electroshock therapy, and the emotional stimuli of fear, panic, and anxiety.

Drug reactions causing neutrophilia are caused by catecholamines, corticosteroids, and others.

The catabolic disorders causing neutrophilia are diabetic acidosis, acute gout, thyroiditis, uremia, Cushing's syndrome, and a few hereditary conditions such as familial neutrophilia.

Eosinophilic leukocytosis

In eosinophilic leukocytosis most of the cells causing the elevated WBC count are eosinophils. Anywhere from 5% up to 90% can be seen, although the most frequently encountered pattern in eosinophilic leukocytosis is an eosinophil count of approximately 10% to 20%. The associated diseases are the following:

1. The most common causes of an increase in eosinophils are allergic disorders of nearly any kind, such as hay fever, asthma, angioneurotic edema, and serum sickness.

2. Parasitic diseases should be considered second in commonality to allergic condi-

tions. *Trichinella* predominates in the United States. Malaria and amebiasis are also possibilities, particularly in view of widespread travel. *Ascaris* is the most common parasite in middle eastern countries. Other parasites associated with eosinophilia are ameba, hookworm, schistosoma, and toxoplasma. In making the differential diagnosis of eosinophilic leukocytosis, particularly when parasites are a consideration, the epidemiology of the suspected disease and the area in which the patient has traveled become of prime importance.

3. Other rarer conditions associated with mild to moderate eosinophilia are malignant conditions such as mycosis fungoides, brain tumors, Hodgkin's disease, and other lymphomas. Gastrointestinal causes include colitis and protein-losing enteropathy. In hypoadrenocorticism, eosinophilia may be found and may suggest the diagnosis of Addison's disease if other features of the disease are found.

4. An extremely high eosinophil count in the range of 80% to 90% usually indicates eosinophilic granulomatosis or eosinophilic leukemia.

Basophilic leukocytosis

An elevated WBC count associated with basophilia is uncommon and most frequently suggests some kind of myeloproliferative disease such as myelofibrosis, agnogenic myeloid metaplasia, and polycythemia vera. A rapid fall in the basophil count may herald an anaphylactic reaction.

Lymphocytosis

Lymphocytosis may be mild to severe and occurs in two varieties: relative, in which the total number of circulating lymphocytes is unchanged but the WBC count is low because of neutropenia; and absolute, in which the number of circulating lymphocytes increases. Relative lymphocytosis accompanies most conditions mentioned in the section on leukopenia associated with neutropenia.

The most common cause of severe lymphocytosis, 80% to 90% mature lymphocytes, is chronic lymphocytic leukemia. This is associated with a marked elevation of the leukocyte count.

Marked lymphocytosis with moderate leukocytosis is found in infectious diseases, particularly pertussis, infectious mononucleosis, and acute infectious lymphocytosis.

Mild to moderate relative lymphocytosis is seen mainly in viral infections with exanthema such as measles, rubella, chicken pox, and roseola infantum.

In bacterial infections, mild to moderate lymphocytosis associated with mild to moderate leukocytosis usually indicates a chronic infectious state. Depending on the overall presenting picture other considerations are brucellosis, typhoid and paratyphoid fever, and chronic granulomatous diseases such as tuberculosis.

In noninfectious disorders and nonmyeloproliferative diseases, thyrotoxicosis and adrenal insufficiency (Addison's disease) are associated with mild to moderate lymphocytosis.

Relative lymphocytosis is a normal occurrence in children and newborns between 4 months and 4 years of age.

RED BLOOD CELL COUNT (RBC)

Red blood cells (erythrocytes) are formed in the red bone marrow. Their production (erythropoiesis) is inhibited by a rise in the circulating red cell level and stimulated by anemia and hypoxia. The hormone erythropoietin mediates the responses to these normal and abnormal situations. (Tissue hypoxia is the ultimate stimulus for erythropoietin production.)

The red blood cells contain a complex compound called hemoglobin, which is made up of heme, a pigmented compound containing iron, and globin, a colorless protein. Hemoglobin binds with oxygen (a reversible reaction) and can also combine with carbon dioxide. Thus, the red blood cell functions primarily to transport oxygen to the tissues and to carry carbon dioxide to the lungs.

The red blood cell (RBC) count represents the number of RBCs in one microliter of whole blood. The correct RBC count can be obtained by multiplying the figure obtained from the automated Coulter counter by one million. For example, an RBC count reported to be 5.11 should be interpreted as 5,110,000 RBCs in one microliter of blood.

In the past, the determination of the red blood cell count was tedious and occasionally erroneous. Thus, the determination of the hematocrit and hemoglobin were adopted for routine use. However, because of the development of automated methods, particularly the Coulter counter, routine hematologic determinations are now quick and accurate. The RBC count is, however, still not used as much as the hemoglobin and hematocrit determinations, which are also part of the Coulter panel.

Normal RBC count

The normal RBC count is between 4.6 and 6.2 $\times$ 10^6 per microliter for men, and between 4.2 and 5.4 $\times$ 10^6 per microliter for women.

The main value of the RBC count is a routine screening examination lies in the gross evaluation of the indices, which are also obtained through automated means, either directly through a writeout from the Coulter counter or through the automatic analyzer.

The erythrocyte indices

The relationship between the number, size, and hemoglobin content of the RBCs is important in accurately describing anemias. An index of these elements may be obtained from an inspection of the stained peripheral blood smear.

Terminology (the peripheral blood smear)

Hematocrit (Hct) is the volume of packed red blood cells found in 100 ml of blood. For example, a value of 46% implies that there are 46 ml of red blood cells in 100 ml of blood. The normal Hct in the male is 40% to 54%; in the female it is 38% to 47%.

Hemoglobin (Hgb) is the oxygen-carrying pigment of the red blood cells and is reported in grams per 100 ml. For example, a value of 15.5 implies that there are 15.5 gm of hemoglobin in each 100 ml of blood. The normal hemoglobin in the male is 13.5 to 18.0 gm/ml; in the female it is 12.0 to 16.0 gm/ml.

Mean cell volume (MCV) describes the red cells in terms of individual cell size. It is given usually as a direct writeout from the automated system. However, it can also be calculated by dividing the volume of packed cells (hematocrit) by the number of RBCs. The result is expressed as microcubic millimeters per red cell. The normal MCV is 82 to 98 cu microns.

Mean cell hemoglobin concentration (MCHC) measures the concentration of hemoglobin in grams per 100 ml of RBCs. This can be done by dividing the hemoglobin in grams by the hematocrit. The percentage is obtained by multiplying this figure by 100. The normal MCHC is 32% to 36%.

Mean cell hemoglobin (MCH) is the hemoglobin content of each individual red blood cell and is calculated by dividing the hemoglobin by the red blood cell count. It is expressed as micromicrograms or picograms of hemoglobin per red blood cell. The normal MCH is 27 to 31 pg.

Examining the peripheral smear

Platelets. Platelets are important in blood coagulation and are visible on stained blood smears. Their absolute absence from the peripheral smear is extremely significant indicating an aplastic bone marrow. Decreased number of platelets (thrombocytopenia) may be caused by various etiologies.

Sometimes a careful observation of the peripheral smear is a better indication of the platelet status than is an absolute platelet count. This observation is easy to do, quick, and accurate. The shape and character of the platelets are also important. When an abnormality is noted it is termed thrombocytopathy (abnormal-looking thrombocytes). Thrombocytosis is the term used when there is an unusually large number of platelets in the blood. This will be seen most often in the blood smear of polycythemia, in a splenectomy status, and in essential thrombocytosis.

Polycythemia

Polycythemia is any condition in which the number of circulating erythrocytes rises above normal. When the red cell mass increases in response to an identifiable physiologic or pathologic stimulus, the condition is called secondary polycythemia. If no etiology can be documented, the change is considered primary, and is described as polycythemia vera (true polycythemia).

Polycythemia vera, according to some authorities, is equivalent to leukemia and in some cases does progress into one of the myeloproliferative diseases.

Secondary polycythemia has been found in erythropoietin-secreting tumors, hypernephroma, renal cysts, and hepatic carcinoma. It has also been associated with chronic obstructive pulmonary disease or cyanotic congenital heart disease with hypoxemia, and is accompanied by an elevated erythropoietin level.

Erythropoietin, a hormone thought to be formed by the action of a renal factor on a plasma globulin, stimulates the proliferation and release of RBCs from the bone marrow into the peripheral circulation. One of the most sensitive ways of differentiating between primary and secondary polycythemia is the determination of the erythropoietin level. This level is diminished in polycythemia vera because the excess number of RBCs produced in this disease suppresses the production of the hormone. The level is elevated in secondary polycythemia.

Normal absolute RBC count and the peripheral smear

Findings on the blood film may suggest a disorder when the absolute RBC count is within normal limits, such as may occur in the following:
1. Significant spherocytosis, polychromatophilia, and erythrocyte agglutination suggest compensated, acquired hemolytic anemia.
2. Spherocytosis with polychromatophilia is very suggestive of hereditary spherocytosis.
3. Target cells are found mainly in hemoglobin C disease.
4. Marked hypochromia associated with target cells is suggestive of thalassemia major or thalessemia minor.
5. Erythrocytes with basophilic stipplings are characteristic of lead poisoning.
6. Macrocytosis in association with hypersegmented neutrophils suggests vitamin B_{12} and/or folic acid deficiency.
7. Rouleaux formation suggests multiple myeloma or macroglobulinemia.
8. Parasites in RBCs are the distinguishing characteristic of malaria.
9. Schistocytes and "burr" cells in association with a decreased platelet count suggest consumption coagulopathy.
10. Mechanical hemolysis is suggested by schistocytes and "burr" cells.
11. A relative increase in neutrophils with increased band forms and toxic granulations suggests severe infection.
12. Atypical lymphocytes indicate the possibility of infectious mononucleosis.
13. Decreased neutrophils and increased lymphocytes suggest agranulocytosis.
14. Eosinophilia usually suggests an allergic reaction.
15. Blast (primitive) forms indicate the possibility of acute leukemia.

Anemia

Anemia is a deficiency of the total hemoglobin red cell mass and is the result of many disorders. Usually anemias are classified into three broad categories:
1. Hypochromic microcytic anemia
2. Normochromic normocytic anemia
3. Macrocytic normochromic, hypochromic, or hyperchromic anemia

Terminology

normochromic normal color (normal hemoglobin content)
hypochromic less than normal color (decreased hemoglobin content)
hyperchromic more than normal color (increased hemoglobin content)
normocytic normal cell size
microcytic smaller than normal cell size
macrocytic larger than normal cell size

Hypochromic microcytic anemia

Iron deficiency. The most frequent cause of hypochromic microcytic anemia is iron deficiency. The patient may or may not have an overt anemia. However, a borderline low hematocrit and hemoglobin, even though the RBC count is normal, should suggest the possibility of hypochromic microcytic anemia. Although the number of cells may be within normal limits, there is a definite dimunition in the size of the RBCs as well as in the hemoglobin concentration.

The hemoglobinopathies. This term is used to describe the clinical syndromes produced in persons having production of abnormal types of hemoglobin resulting from genetic reasons. The most important of these syndromes are thalassemia major and thalassemia minor (Mediterranean anemia), sickle cell anemia, and hemoglobin C disease. The blood picture of the hemoglobinopathies simulates that of iron deficiency anemia on the peripheral smear. However, the bone marrow stores, serum iron level, and iron binding capacity will differentiate between the two.

Normochromic normocytic anemia

The most common cause of normocytic normochromic anemia is an acute loss of red blood cell mass such as occurs in hemorrhage or hemolysis.

Hypoplastic anemia

Another major group of normochromic normocytic anemias are the aplastic or hypoplastic anemias. In some very rare situations a combination of macrocytic and microcytic anemia may produce a normal index. Such a situation will occur in vitamin B_{12} deficiency anemia associated with carcinoma of the stomach and chronic blood loss. However, the overall clinical picture and other clues on the blood smear (multi-segmented leukocytes and mild hemolysis) will suggest pathology.

Macrocytic anemia

In macrocytic anemia there is a decreased absolute number of RBCs per cubic micrometer. However, the individual cells are larger in diameter and volume and contain more hemoglobin than normal. Consequently, there will be an elevated MCV and MCHC.

The two most common diseases associated with macrocytosis with significant anemia are folic acid deficiency and vitamin B_{12} deficiency, which is also known as Addisonian or pernicious anemia. These two conditions are also associated with megaloblastic changes in the bone marrow.

Some macrocytosis is also observed in the anemia of myxedema, as well as in the anemias following acute blood loss, either through bleeding or hemolysis. The latter two conditions are not accompanied by megaloblastic changes in the bone marrow since the macrocytosis reflects increased reticulocytes, which are slightly larger than normal RBCs.

Macrocytic normochromic anemia is also seen in some cases of chronic liver disease, hypothyroidism, and aplastic anemia.

Sedimentation rate (sed rate or ESR)

The sedimentation rate is the speed with which RBCs settle in uncoagulated blood. This rate is affected by many factors, too numerous to mention in this book. It is, therefore, a nonspecific test, having neither organ nor disease specificity. Its chief value lies in the fact that a normal value does diminish the probability of a significant disease process, giving some reassurance to the investigator. An abnormal result indicates that a more extensive search is necessary.

In addition to its general screening value, the sed rate is useful in following the progress of certain diseases such as rheumatic fever. A gradually diminishing sed rate indicates a better prognosis, whereas a gradually increasing rate indicates a poorer prognosis.

NORMAL SEDIMENTATION RATE (WESTERGREN)

Men under 50 yrs: <15 mm/hr
Men over 50 yrs: <20 mm/hr
Women under 50 yrs: <20 mm/hr
Women over 50 yrs: <30 mm/hr

CHAPTER 3

Urinalysis

The urine examination, properly performed, may give valuable information.

The urine that is to be analyzed should be a clean catch (midstream) specimen collected in a clean, dry container and examined as quickly as possible, preferably within two hours. It should be a morning specimen and the patient should not have had fluids for twelve hours preceding the collection of the urine. Urine becomes alkaline on standing, bacteria multiply, and leukocytes and casts disintegrate.

The standard urinalysis includes pH, specific gravity, the presence or absence of glucose and ketones, protein semiquantitation, and microscopic examination of the centrifuged urinary sediment.

pH (ACIDITY OR ALKALINITY)

Normal fresh urine is usually acid, with a pH of 4.6 to 8. If the specimen has not been standing too long, the pH will reflect the patient's acid-base balance.

An alkaline urine is seen in metabolic alkalosis. The exception to this is long-standing hypokalemic chloremic alkalosis, in which a potassium deficiency causes the renal tubular cells to secrete hydrogen ions in lieu of potassium. A paradoxical aciduria is the result. This situation (metabolic alkalosis with aciduria) may suggest generalized intracellular acidosis.

SPECIFIC GRAVITY (S.G.)

NORMAL SPECIFIC GRAVITY

1.016-1.022 (normal fluid intake)
1.001-1.035 (range)

The specific gravity of a morning urine specimen voided by a fasting patient reflects the maximum concentrating ability of the kidney. In the absence of formed elements, protein, or glycosuria, the specific gravity in a clear urine should be 1.025 to 1.030. Anything below this value reflects distal renal tubular disease and inability of the kidney to concentrate urine to the maximum. Endocrine disease associated with insufficient ADH secretion is also a possibility.

A fixed specific gravity indicates chronic glomerulopyelonephritis.

A long-standing hypokalemic and hypercalcemic nephropathy, in which the patient has symptoms of frequency, nocturia, and polyuria can be easily diagnosed by a proper examination of the urine for specific gravity and osmolality. The specimen should be collected after overnight fasting. If simultaneous serum and urine osmolality determinations are performed, the serum osmolality will be high while the urine osmolality will be relatively low.

GLUCOSE

When a urine specimen voided in the morning is free of glucose, diabetes mellitus is not ruled out because, normally, a blood sugar of 130 to 140 mg/100 ml is necessary before traces of glucose appear in the urine.

Glucosuria means one of two things: diabetes mellitus or a low renal threshold for glucose resorption if the blood glucose level is normal.

PROTEIN

The absence of protein in the urine, particularly in a concentrated urine, rules out significant renal glomerular disease. The presence of protein in the urine indicates the possibility of any one of a large number of diseases, the differential diagnosis of which will be discussed in Chapter 6, pp. 114-119.

When there is a trace of protein in the urine, a follow-up is indicated. However, if there is more than a trace, twenty-four-hour urine excretion of protein should be ascertained. For a more specific diagnosis, a quantitative analysis of the kind of protein, be it albumin, one of the globulins, or Bence Jones proteins, should be performed.

MICROSCOPIC EXAMINATION OF SEDIMENT

Normally, a microscopic examination of the sediment in the urine will show fewer than one or two RBCs, one or two WBCs, and only an occasional cast. Anything more is considered pathologic. Urine microscopy is especially important in making the diagnosis of acute pyelonephritis, the classical findings of which are numerous WBCs, WBC casts, and bacteria.

Casts

Casts are formed in the kidney tubules by the agglutination of protein cells, or cellular debris. Their presence in the urine implies tubular or glomerular disorders. Because casts are cylindrical structures, their occurrence in the urine is sometimes called cylindruria. Since protein is necessary for cast formation, proteinuria often accompanies cylindruria.

WBC casts indicate pyelonephritis, and sometimes are also found in the exudative stage of acute glomerulonephritis. RBC casts may appear colorless if only a few RBCs are present. However, they are often yellow. Their presence indicates glomerulo-nephritis.

Epithelial casts may be difficult to distinguish from leukocyte or mixed-cell casts. When they are seen together with red blood cells and lipids in the casts, glomerulo-nephritis is suggested.

A coarsely granular cast is the result of the first step in the disintegration of the WBC or epithelial cell cast. If disintegration continues, the coarse granules break down to small granules, forming the finely granular cast. The next step is the formation of what is known as the waxy cast, which is translucent and shaped by the tubule where it was formed.

Hyaline casts are clear, colorless cylinders made up of protein. They pass almost unchanged down the tubules. They may be coarsely or finely granular depending upon the degenerative changes that took place in the tubules. The appearance of hyaline casts alone is usually a sudden, mild, and temporary phenomenon and must be correlated with other clinical findings.

Urine that is loaded with hyaline casts and protein is suggestive of the nephrotic syndrome, since they are seen in concentrated acid urine high in protein.

Red blood cells

The appearance of red blood cells in the urine is an indication of bleeding after the blood has passed through the glomeruli and tubules, such as would occur with hemorrhagic cystitis or calculi in the renal pelvis. Another possibility would be disease of the renal collecting and tubular systems, such as tuberculosis or tumors.

Telescoping

Urine sediment that shows different stages of glomerular nephritis (acute and subacute) and that also has the findings of the nephrotic syndrome is called "telescoping" of the urine. Such a sediment is seen in lupus nephritis.

Crystals

The type of crystals found in normal urine varies with the pH of the specimen. Calcium oxalate, uric acid, and urate crystals may be seen in acid urine. Phosphate and carbonate crystals and amorphous phosphates are often seen in alkaline urine.

Calcium oxalate crystals, if numerous, may suggest hypercalcemia.

APPEARANCE

The color of the urine is not usually reported in the routine urinalysis and should be specifically requested if a rare diagnosis is suspected.

The normal urine is golden yellow. A darker color suggests hematuria, hemo-globinuria, bilirubinuria, urobilinuria, or porphyria. Tests specifically directed toward the cause of these entities should be ordered.

A urine that changes to a bright burgundy red when exposed to the light is highly suggestive of porphyria.

Tea-colored urine that stains the underwear indicates the possibility of obstructive jaundice with urobilinogen in the urine.

The fruity aroma of a diabetic urine and the red discoloration of the urine in patients taking pyridium are two well-known diagnostic clues commonly encountered in the emergency room.

Common variances in the routine screening panel and clinical implications

This appendix contains some of the most common variances found in the routine screening examination and the clinical implications or potential disease condition that may exist. Generally speaking, a variance in one value has more significance when compared with the results of the total examination.

This appendix has been provided so that the reader can more easily determine what further action is indicated when there is a variance from a normal value. The last column refers the reader to the page on which are found additional tests for the evaluation or confirmation of a suspected disease condition.

BLOOD CHEMISTRY

Test	Abbreviation	Normal value	Variance	Clinical implication	Subsequent laboratory studies, comments, and/or conclusive symptoms
Alkaline phosphatase (total serum)	alk phos	Adults: 1.5-4.5 U/dll (Bodansky) 4-13 U/ml (King-Armstrong) 0.8-2.3 U/ml (Bessey-Lowry) 15-35 U/ml (Shinowara-Jones-Reinhart) Children: 5.0-14.0 U/dll (Bodansky) 3.4-9.0 U/ml (Bessey-Lowry) 15-30 U/dll (King-Armstrong)	↑ (marked) with liver disease (bilirubinemia)	Early obstructive jaundice	p. 135
			↑ (marked) without liver disease	Paget's disease of bone	Bone x ray
			↑ (marked)	Carcinoma with bone metastasis	p. 149
			↑ (moderate) with liver disease	Cholangeolitic hepatitis	p. 136
			↑ (mild) with liver disease	Liver cirrhosis with active hepatiti	p. 136
			↑ (mild) without liver disease and with hypercalcemia	Hyperparathyroidism	p. 149
			↑ (mild to moderate) with N or ↓ Ca	Osteomalacia	History, physical, and x rays
Bilirubin (serum)		Up to 0.3 mg/dl (direct or conjugated) 0.1-1.0 mg/dl (indirect or unconjugated) Total: 0.1-1.2 mg/dl Newborn total: 1-12 mg/dl	↑ indirect or unconjugated, with reticulocytes, absent urine bilirubin	Low grade hemolytic disease	p. 136
			↑ indirect or unconjugated with normal liver function	Gilbert's disease	p. 136
			↑ direct or conjugated with abnormal albumin, globulin and enzymes	Parenchymal liver disease, obstructive liver disease	p. 136
			↑ (marked) indirect or unconjugated	Massive hemolysis	p. 136
			↑ (marked) direct or conjugated	Obstructive jaundice: obstructive phase of hepatitis, cholangeitis, lower biliary tract obstruction (carcinoma or calculus)	p. 136

Calcium (serum)	Ca	Ionized: 4.2-5.2 mg/dl 2.1-2.6 mEq/L or 50-58% of total Total: 9.0-10.6 mg/dl 4.5-5.3 mEq/L Infants: 11-13 mg/dl	N with marked ↓ albumin		
			N with ↑ BUN	Hypercalcemia Primary hyperparathyroidism, secondary hyperparathyroidism	See hypercalcemia p. 149
			↑ with ↓ phosphorus and N BUN	Hyperparathyroidism	p. 149
			↑ with ↑ gamma globulin	Sarcoidosis, multiple myeloma, malignancies with possible metastasis to bone	pp. 101, 149, 160
			↑ with metabolic alkalosis	Milk-alkali syndrome	History of peptic ulcer disease
			↑	Severe thyrotoxicosis	pp. 145, 180
			↑	Malignant tumors with or without bone metastasis	p. 149
			↑	Bone fractures	History, physical, and x rays
			↑ with ↑ alk phos	Paget's disease of bone	p. 13
			↓ with ↓ albumin fraction of serum protein	Pseudohypocalcemia	p. 5
			↓ with ↑ phosphorus, N BUN, N creat	Hypoparathyroidism	p. 149
			↓	Osteomalacia (adults), rickets (children)	History, physical, and x rays
			↓	Malabsorption syndrome	p. 128
			↓	Acute pancreatitis	p. 129
			↓	Pregnancy	History and physical
			↓	Diuretics	History
			↓	Respiratory alkalosis	pp. 99, 104
Carbon dioxide combining power (plasma or serum, venous)	CO_2 combining power	24-30 mM/L	↑ without chronic obstructive lung disease and frequently with K and Cl	Hypokalemic-chloremic alkalosis (serum alkalosis and intracellular acidosis)	pp. 99, 104

Continued.

N = normal
↑ = elevated
↓ = depressed

BLOOD CHEMISTRY—cont'd

Test	Abbreviation	Normal value	Variance	Clinical implication	Subsequent laboratory studies, comments, and/or conclusive symptoms
Carbon dioxide combining power—cont'd			→ → →	Uremic acidosis Diabetic ketoacidosis Lactic acidosis	pp. 99, 104 Glucose tolerance test Serum lactic acid levels
			↓ with ↓ K and ↑Cl ↓	Renal tubular acidosis Respiratory alkalosis (hyperventilation syndrome)	pp. 17, 104 pp. 99, 104 (blood pH)
Chloride	Cl	95-103 mEq/L	↑ with ↓ CO_2 combining power and ↓ K	Renal tubular acidosis, iatrogenic (tube feeding and inappropriate IV fluids)	pp. 17, 104
			↓ with ↑CO_2 combining power, and N K	Potassium-saving diuretics	History
			↓ with ↓ K and ↑CO_2 combining power	Hypokalemic-chloremic alkalosis	pp. 99, 104
Cholesterol (total serum)	Chol	150-250 mg/dl (varies with diet and age)	↑ (marked) with ↑ alk phos and ↑ bilirubin	Liver disease with biliary obstruction	p. 136
			↑ (marked) with ↑ BUN and ↑ creat	Nephrotic stage of glomerulonephritis	p. 116
			↑ (marked)	Familial hypercholesterolemia	p. 75
			↓ (marked)	Diet and malnutrition	History and physical
			↓ (marked)	Extensive liver disease	p. 136
			↓ (marked)	Hyperthyroidism	p. 145
Creatinine	Creat	0.6-1.2 mg/dl	↑	Kidney disease with >50% destruction of nephrons	p. 110
Blood glucose	Gluc	70-110 mg/dl	↑	Diabetes mellitus	History and glucose tolerance test
		60-100 mg/dl	↑(mild) with ↑ blood catecholamines	Acute stress, pheochromocytoma	History; p. 155
			↑(mild) with ↑ glucocorticoids	Cushing's syndrome (hyperadrenalism), Cushing's disease (secondary hyperadrenalism)	p. 152

Test	Normal values	Variance	Clinical implication	Reference
		↑ (mild) with ↓ cholesterolemia	Hyperthyroidism	p. 145
		↑ (mild)	Diuretics	History, p. 128
		↑ (mild)	Acute and chronic pancreatic insufficiency	
		↑ (moderate)	Diabetes mellitus	History and glucose tolerance test
		↑ (marked) with ↓ CO_2 combining power	Uncontrolled diabetes and ketoacidosis	Electrolytes
		↑ (marked) with N CO_2 combining power and hypernatremia	Nonketotic, nonacidotic hyperglycemia	Electrolytes
		↓	Pancreatic islet cell tumor	p. 9
		↓	Large nonpancreatic tumor	IVP, laminograms, and KUB
		↓	Pituitary hypofunction	p. 156
		↓ with hyperkalemia, hyponatremia, and ↑ BUN	Addison's disease (adrenocortical hypofunction)	p. 152
		↓	Extensive liver disease	p. 136
		↓	Reactive hypoglycemia	5-hour glucose tolerance test, p. 76
Lactic dehydrogenase (serum)	80-120 Wacker units 150-450 Wroblewski units 71-207 I.U./L	↑ (marked)	Myocardial infarction	p. 57
		↑ (marked)	Hemolytic disorders (pernicious anemia)	p. 59
		↑ (mild)	Chronic viral hepatitis	p. 136
		↑ (mild)	Pneumonia, pulmonary emboli	Chest x ray, p. 105
		↑ (mild)	Generalized viral infections	p. 7
		↑ (mild)	Low grade hemolytic disorders	p. 149
		↑ (mild)	Cerebral vascular accident	p. 171 (spinal tap)
		↑ (mild)	Renal tissue destruction	p. 110
Phosphorus (serum)	Adults: 1.8-2.6 mEq/L 3.0-4.5 mg/dl	↑ with ↑ BUN, ↑ creat	Chronic glomerular disease	p. 110
		↑ with ↓ Ca, N BUN, N creat	Hypoparathyroidism	p. 149

N = normal
↑ = elevated
↓ = depressed

Continued.

BLOOD CHEMISTRY—cont'd

Test	Abbreviation	Normal value	Variance	Clinical implication	Subsequent laboratory studies, comments, and/or conclusive symptoms
Phosphorus—cont'd		Children: 2.3–4.1 mEq/L 4.0–7.0 mg/dl	N or ↑ with N BUN, N creat	Milk-alkali syndrome	History of peptic ulcer disease
			N with ↑Ca and ↑gamma globulin	Sarcoidosis	p. 101
			↓ with ↑Ca, N BUN, N creat	Hyperparathyroidism	p. 149
			↓ with N or ↓ Ca and ↑ alk phos	Rickets (children), osteomalacia (adults)	History, physical, and x rays pp. 17, 104
			→	Renal tubular acidosis	p. 128
			→	Malabsorption syndrome	p. 128
Potassium (plasma)	K	3.8–5.0 mEq/L	↑ with hypovolemia and ↑BUN	Renal failure	p. 110
			↑	Addison's disease	p. 152
			N with ↓ total body K and ↑CO_2 combining power	Chronic diuretic use, alkalosis	History, pp. 99, 104
			↓ with ↑ CO_2 combining power	Cushing's syndrome	p. 152
			→	Primary and secondary hyperaldosteronism with chronic congestive heart failure	History and physical, pp. 76, 154
			→	Liver disease with ascites	History and physical, p. 136
			→	Excessive licorice ingestion (hypertension)	History
			→	Antinflammatory drugs	History
			→	Malignant hypertension, hypertensive disease, unilateral renal vascular hypertension	↑reninemia, p. 154
			→	Poor diet	History
			→	Chronic stress	History
			→	Chronic diarrhea	History
			→	Malabsorption syndrome	p. 128

Test	Abbrev.	Normal values	Variance	Clinical implications	Action/reference
Total protein and albumin/globulin ratio (serum)	Tot prot and A/G ratio	Total: 6.0-7.8 gm/dl Albumin: 3.2-4.5 gm/dl Globulin: 2.3-3.5 gm/dl	↑	Diaphoresis	History
			→	Chronic fever	History and physical
			↓ with ↑Cl and ↓CO_2 combining power	Renal tubular acidosis	p. 104
			↓ with ↓ albumin (<2.5 gm) and ↑ globulin (3 gm) (reversed A/G ratio)	Chronic liver disease	p. 136
			N with ↓ albumin and ↑ globulin (reversed A/G ratio)	Myeloproliferative diseases, chronic granulomatous infectious diseases	Serum protein electrophoresis, p. 159
Sodium (serum)	Na	136-142 mEq/L	↑	Iatrogenic	History
			↑ with hyperglycemia	Hypothalamic lesion, head trauma, and hyperosmolar states	History and physical
			↓ with dehydration (slight ↑ BUN)	Addison's disease (primary adrenocortical deficiency)	p. 152
			↓ with N or ↑ BUN	Chronic sodium-losing nephropathy	pp. 17, 110
			↓ with ↓Cl	Vomiting, diarrhea or tube drainage	History
			→	Diaphoresis, burns	History and physical
			→	Diuretics (mercurial and chlorothiazide)	History
			↓ with ↑ BUN, ↑ creat	Chronic renal insufficiency with acidosis	pp. 17, 104
			→	Starvation with acidosis, diabetic acidosis	pH
			→	Paracentesis, thoracentesis	History
			→	Dilution hyponatremia: diuretics with Na restriction, secondary hyperaldosteronism, hepatic failure with ascites, congestive heart failure, excessive water administration, acute or chronic renal insufficiency (oliguria), hypothermia, lobar pneumonia	History and physical, pp. 76, 78, 110, 136

N = normal
↑ = elevated
↓ = depressed

Continued.

BLOOD CHEMISTRY—cont'd

Test	Abbreviation	Normal value	Variance	Clinical implication	Subsequent laboratory studies, comments, and/or conclusive symptoms
Sodium—cont'd			↓ with inappropriate ADH syndrome (↑ S.G. and ↓ Na)	Bronchogenic carcinoma, pulmonary infections, and porphyria	Chest x ray
Serum glutamic oxaloacetic transaminase	SGOT	8-33 U/ml	↑ (marked)	Acute severe fulminating hepatitis, severe liver necrosis, and acute myocardial infarction	pp. 57, 136
			↑ (moderate)	Myocarditis, cardiomyopathies	p. 57
			↑ (mild)	Cirrhosis, cholangiolitic jaundice, metastatic liver disease, skeletal muscle disease, posttrauma, and generalized infections, dissecting aneurysm, pulmonary infarction, shock, pericarditis	p. 136, history and physical
Blood urea nitrogen	BUN	8-18 mg/dl	↑	Acute or chronic renal failure, congestive heart failure with decreased renal blood supply, and obstructive uropathy	pp. 76, 110
Uric acid (serum)		Male: 2.1-7.8 mg/dl Female: 2.0-6.4 mg/dl	↑ with acute arthritis	Gout	X ray and twenty-four-hour urine excretion of uric acid
			↑ (mild)	Idiopathic	
			↑ with ↑ BUN, ↑ creat	Chronic renal failure	p. 110
			↑	Starvation	History and physical
			↑	Glycogen storage disease	Liver biopsy or bone marrow biopsy
			↑	Diuretics	History

N = normal   ↑ = elevated   ↓ = depressed

HEMATOLOGY

Test	Abbreviation	Normal value	Variance	Clinical implication	Subsequent laboratory studies, comments, and/or conclusive symptoms
White blood cell count	WBC	4500-11,000/microliter	↑(mild to moderate)	Infectious disease, mainly bacterial and moderate	History, physical, and differential
			↑(mild to moderate)	Severe sepsis in elderly patients	History, physical, and differential
			↑(marked)	Severe sepsis	History, physical, and differential
Red blood cell count	RBC	Male: $4.6\text{-}6.2 \times 10^6$/microliter Female: $4.2\text{-}5.4 \times 10^6$/microliter	↑(primary)	Polycythemia vera (leukemia)	↓erythropoietin level
			↑(secondary)	Chronic obstructive lung disease, cyanotic congenital heart diseases with hypoxemia	p. 97 and ↑erythropoietin level
The differential WBC count					
Neutrophils		Mean %: 56% Range of absolute counts: 1800-7000/microliter	↑(mild to moderate)	Bacterial infections, inflammatory disorders, tumors, physical and emotional stimuli, stresses (heat, extreme cold, exercise, electroshock therapy, emotional stimuli), and drugs (catecholamines, corticosteroids)	History and physical, and cultures
			↓(mild to moderate) with monocytosis (up to 50%)	Familial benign neutropenia	History

Continued.

N = normal
↑ = elevated
↓ = depressed

HEMATOLOGY—cont'd

Test	Abbreviation	Normal value	Variance	Clinical implication	Subsequent laboratory studies, comments, and/or conclusive symptoms
Neutrophils—cont'd			↓ (mild to moderate)	Acute viral infections, anorexia nervosa (starvation), primary and secondary splenic neutropenia, drug induced, and acute alcoholic ingestion	History and physical
Eosinophils		Mean %: 2.7%	↑	Allergic disorders, parasitic diseases	History and physical, p. 129
		Range of absolute counts: 0–450/microliter	↑ (90%)	Eosinophilic leukemia	p. 29
			↑ ↓	Acute and chronic stress (emotional or somatic), Endocrine causes (excess ACTH, cortisone, epinephrine, intermenstrual period, diurnal variations, and acromegaly)	History, p. 141
Basophils		Mean %: 0.3%	↑	Myeloproliferative disease	p. 29
		Range of absolute counts: 0–200/microliter	↓	Anaphylactic reaction	Serology
			↓ with granulocytopenia	Acute hypersensitive reactions, steroids, diurnal changes, hyperthyroidism, pituitary basophilism, radiation therapy, acute and chronic infection, ovulation, pregnancy, and aging	History and physical, p. 27
Lymphocytes		Mean %: 34%	↑ (80%-90%) with ↑ (marked) leukocytes	Chronic lymphocytic leukemia	p. 29
		Range of absolute counts: 1000–4800/microliter	↑ (marked) with ↑ (moderate) leukocytes	Infectious diseases: pertussis, infectious mononucleosis, and acute infectious lymphocytosis	pp. 33, 159, 182 (bone marrow, peripheral smear)
			↑ (mild to moderate relative) In bacterial infections: ↑ (mild to moderate) with ↑ (mild to moderate) leukocytes	Viral infections with eczemas	History and physical
				Chronic infectious state	History and physical

The peripheral smear

	Normal value	Variance	Clinical implication	Reference
Platelets	290,000/mm (140,000-440,000) Brecher-Cronkite method	↑ (mild to moderate) in noninfectious and nonmyeloproliferative disease	Thyrotoxicosis, adrenal insufficiency (Addison's disease)	pp. 145, 152
		Absolute absence	Aplastic bone marrow, thrombocytopenia (various etiologies)	p. 159
		↑	Polycythemia, splenectomy status, essential thrombocytosis	p. 20, ↓hemopoietin, history
Hemoglobin Hgb	Male: 13.5-18.0 gm/dl Female: 12.0-16.0 gm/dl	↓	Anemia	p. 159
		↓ (borderline) with ↓ (borderline) Hct and N RBC count	Hypochromic microcytic anemia: iron deficiency, thalassemia major and minor, sickle cell anemia, and hemoglobin C disease	p. 159 (bone marrow), ↓ serum iron level, Hgb electrophoresis, p. 164
		↓	Normochromic normocytic anemia	History, reticulocyte count
		↓ with ↑ MCV and ↑ MCHC	Macrocytic anemia: folic acid deficiency, vitamin B_{12} deficiency (pernicious anemia)	pp. 159, 166

Additional findings on the peripheral smear

		Spherocytosis, polychromatophilia, and erythrocyte agglutination	Compensated, acquired hemolytic anemia	p. 165
		Spherocytosis with polychromatophilia	Hereditary spherocytosis	p. 165
		Basophilic stipplings	Lead poisoning	Peripheral smear for lead
		Macrocytosis and hypersegmental neutrophils	Vitamin B_{12} and/or folic acid deficiency	p. 159

N = normal
↑ = elevated
↓ = depressed

Continued.

HEMATOLOGY—cont'd

Test	Abbreviation	Normal value	Variance	Clinical implication	Subsequent laboratory studies, comments, and/or conclusive symptoms
Additional findings on the peripheral smear—cont'd					
			Rouleaux formation	Multiple myeloma or macroglobulinemia	p. 160
			Parasites in RBCs	Malaria	p. 32
			Schistocytes and "burr" cells with ↓ platelet count	Consumption coagulopathy	p. 160
			Schistocytes and "burr" cells	Mechanical hemolysis (prostatic valves)	History
			↑ neutrophils, ↑ band forms and toxic granulations	Severe infection	History and physical
			Atypical lymphocytes	Infectious mononucleosis	p. 182
			↓ neutrophils and increased lymphocytes	Agranulocytosis	p. 159
			Eosinophilia	Allergy reaction	History
			Blast (primitive) forms	Acute leukemia	p. 11

N = normal   ↑ = elevated   ↓ = depressed

URINALYSIS

Test	Abbreviation	Normal value	Variance	Clinical implication	Subsequent laboratory studies, comments, and/or conclusive symptoms
pH (acidity or alkalinity)		4.6-8.0	↑ (alkaline) with CO_2 combining power	Metabolic alkalosis	pp. 99, 104
			↓ (aciduria) with metabolic alkalosis, ↓ K, ↓ Cl	Generalized intracellular acidosis	pp. 99, 104
Specific gravity	S.G.	1.016-1.022 (normal fluid intake)	↓ with ↓ K, ↓ Ca, ↑ Cl	Distal renal tubular disease	p. 110
			Fixed S.G. (isosthenuria)	Chronic renal disease	p. 110

			1.001-1.035 (range)	↓ with ↑ Ca, ↓ K	Hypokalemic and hypercalcemic nephropathy	p. 110
Glucose (qualitative)	Gluc		Negative	Glycosuria with ↑ blood glucose	Diabetes mellitus	Gluc tolerance test
				Glycosuria with ↓ blood gluc	Low renal threshold for glucose resorption	Gluc tolerance test
Protein (qualitative)			Negative	Proteinuria (trace)	Follow-up indicated	p. 36
				Proteinuria (more than a trace)	Twenty-four hour urine quantitative analysis indicated	
Microscopic examination						
Casts			Negative	WBC casts	Pyelonephritis	p. 110
				RBC casts	Glomerulonephritis	p. 110
				Hyaline casts with proteinuria	Nephrotic syndrome	p. 116
Red blood cells	RBCs		Negative	Hematuria	Hemorrhagic cystitis or calculi in the renal pelvis, tuberculosis or tumors of the renal collecting and tubular system	p. 110
Crystals			Negative	Present with amorphous substances and ↑ uric acid	Possible gouty nephropathy	p. 51
				Calcium oxalate crystals with ↑ serum calcium	Suggests hypercalcemia	p. 149
Color			Golden yellow	Darker color	Hematuria, bilirubinuria, hemoglobinuria, urobilinuria, and porphyria	pp. 118, 136
				Color changes when exposed to light	Porphyria	p. 37
				Tea-colored and staining (urobilinogen in urine)	Possible obstructive jaundice	p. 136

N = normal
↑ = elevated
↓ = depressed

Evaluative and diagnostic laboratory tests for specific diseases

Unit One dealt with the routine screening of the patient through laboratory tests. In Unit Two additional tests are discussed to provide guidelines in ordering and understanding the tests that will lead to a more definitive diagnosis when an abnormality is detected in the screening examination.

The anatomy and physiology of the organ or system that is involved in the disease process are developed before the specific laboratory tests are discussed so that the rationale behind the test, the nomenclature and the limitations of the specific test may be better understood.

CHAPTER 4

Diagnostic tests for cardiovascular disorders

ANATOMY AND PHYSIOLOGY

The heart is a muscular pump with four chambers guarded by four valves. It is innervated by the autonomic nervous system, receives its blood supply from the coronary arteries, and possesses a marvelous conductive system, which stimulates it to beat and assures adequate conduction velocity.

The course of the blood through the four chambers of the heart and the great vessels is shown in Fig. 4-1. The blood enters the two atria simultaneously, unimpeded by valves. The right atrium receives venous blood through the inferior and superior vena cavae. The left atrium receives arterial blood through the pulmonary veins (4). During diastole both the atria and the ventricles fill. During atrial systole an extra complement of blood is pushed into the ventricles. When ventricular systole begins the two valves (mitral and tricuspid) guarding the atria close (S_1), and blood is pumped to the lungs from the right ventricle via the pulmonary artery and to the systemic circulation from the left ventricle via the aorta. When diastole begins the valves (pulmonary and aortic) guarding the two ventricles close (S_2).

The two coronary arteries (right and left) spring from the root of the aorta. During diastole the coronary arteries fill, supplying the myocardium with oxygenated blood.

The conductive system of the heart is shown in Fig. 4-2. The sinus node paces the heart and lies in the superior portion of the right atrium. The atrioventricular (A-V) node lies in the lower part of the right atrium. Its function is to receive the impulse from the sinus node and delay it slightly so that the atria will have time to pump their contents into the ventricles before they contract, thus complementing cardiac output. The internodal tracts connect the two nodes and ensure rapid conduction velocity between them. The interatrial tract (Bachmann's bundle) speeds the impulse to the left atrium.

Since there is a fibrous ring separating the atria from the ventricles, the bundle of His is the sole muscular connection between these two parts of the heart. The

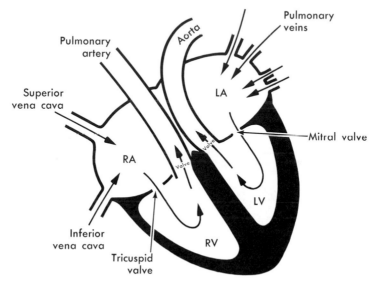

Fig. 4-1. The course of blood flow through the heart chambers and great vessels. (From Zalis, E. G., and Conover, M. H.: Understanding electrocardiography: physiological and interpretive concepts, St. Louis, 1972, The C. V. Mosby Co.)

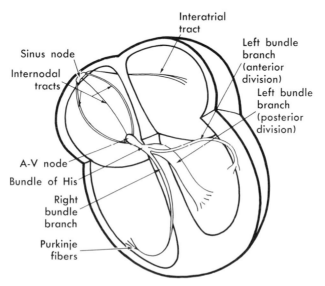

Fig. 4-2. The conductive system.

impulse, then, enters the A-V node and is passed down the bundle of His and rapidly completes its journey through the ventricles via the bundle branches and the Purkinje fibers. The right bundle branch serves the right side of the heart and the left bundle branch, which is divided into an anterior and a posterior division, serves the left side.

The conductive system of the heart enables the impulse to travel six times faster than would be possible without it.

ROUTINE TESTS
The electrocardiogram (ECG)

This brief section on electrocardiography will not teach the performance or interpretation of electrocardiograms. It is hoped that it will increase appreciation of the value and the limits of this diagnostic test and will provide the motivation for a further study of the subject. Subsequent sections will assume a working knowledge of the vocabulary used in electrocardiography. Although the electrocardiogram is used in almost all types of heart disease, this section will emphasize those areas in which the test has been found most useful.

Coronary artery disease

The electrocardiogram is indispensable in the proper diagnosis and treatment of coronary artery disease, and its use extends from the asymptomatic person with a normal resting electrocardiogram (by means of stress electrocardiography, see the section on exercise electrocardiography) to the patient with acute myocardial infarction.

Electrocardiogram changes in coronary artery disease include the following.

ST-T abnormalities. "Nonspecific ST-T abnormalities" is one of the most common electrocardiographic interpretations made. This vague and nonspecific interpretation can frustrate the beginner or one who expects a diagnostic label from every ECG. This is not always possible. Nonspecific ST-T abnormalities are what the term says they are. They are changes of the S-T segment and the T waves that are outside the range of what is considered normal, and this renders the electrocardiogram abnormal. They can be seen in a variety of disorders, cardiac or noncardiac, and do not necessarily signify heart disease. Still, these deviations may be the earliest manifestations of coronary artery disease.

S-T depressions. These may indicate myocardial ischemia and are more specific changes, being flat or downsloping of 1 mm or more. Although not diagnostic of coronary artery disease, they are quite characteristic. Digitalis and electrolyte abnormalities can accentuate or even mimic these changes.

S-T elevations. Marked S-T elevations in well localized leads in a 45-year-old man clutching his chest in the emergency room is the hallmark of acute myocardial infarction. But an unqualified diagnosis of acute myocardial infarction would be incorrect. Such a tracing from the person may reflect early changes in acute myocardial infarction ("hyperacute") or may revert to normal in a matter of minutes, at which time they would be characteristic of Prinzmetal's angina, reflecting massive but totally reversible myocardial ischemia. Thus an unqualified diagnosis of myocardial infarction, either acute or chronic, cannot be based upon an abnormality of ST-T waves, regardless of the severity of the changes. Abnormal Q waves (see the section on QRS changes) are necessary before such a diagnosis is made. S-T elevations that remain unchanged, especially following an acute myocardial infarction, may point to a ventricular aneurysm.

T inversions. Prominent or giant T inversions may reflect diffuse myocardial ischemia or possibly subendocardial infarction but are by no means specific. Among the many causes of T wave inversions are central nervous system lesions, usually due to massive damage or subarachnoid hemorrhage. These conditions can produce marked T wave inversions that can easily be confused with those of severe coronary artery disease.

QRS changes. Changes of the QRS complex are commonly seen in coronary artery disease. Abnormal Q waves are the hallmark of myocardial infarction. By also observing the associated changes in the ST-T segment, one can make a reasonable estimate of the age of the infarction as to acute, subacute, or chronic. It is generally accepted that the more the number of leads in which the Q waves are seen, the larger the infarction. Also, most Q waves persist indefinitely, but it is not uncommon for an electrocardiogram with diagnostic Q waves to lose the Q waves or even revert to normal months or years following an infarction.

Pathologic Q waves do not necessarily signify coronary artery disease or myocardial infarction. They can be seen in other conditions most characteristic of infiltrative myocardial disorders, such as amyloidosis.

P waves. Diagnostic usefulness of the P waves in coronary artery disease is limited. In patients with atrial infarctions or heart failure with elevated pressures in the left atrium, P waves may become abnormal.

U waves. These are seen in normal people, become more prominent in electrolyte disorders (hypokalemia), and may be inverted in myocardial ischemia.

P-R segment. The P-R segment is commonly normal in coronary artery disease. Prolonged P-R segment (first degree heart block) is frequently seen in patients with myocardial infarction, especially of the inferior wall. Prolonged P-R segment also can result from digitalis excess.

Q-T interval. The Q-T interval in coronary artery disease with myocardial ischemia may be prolonged. This fact is helpful in differentiating the ST-T abnormalities due to ischemia (which is accompanied by Q-T prolongation) from those changes caused by digitalis (which is commonly accompanied by Q-T shortening).

Other clinical uses for the ECG

Besides the diagnosis of coronary artery disease, the electrocardiogram is invaluable in the diagnosis of rhythm disorders due to coronary artery disease and in valvular heart disease, in which stenosis or regurgitation of various valves can cause hypertrophy or enlargement of the respective chambers.

Valvular heart disease. Valvular heart disease is commonly reflected in the electrocardiogram by either increased voltage or ST-T abnormalities of the leads reflecting those chambers. Common examples include the following. *Aortic stenosis* or *aortic insufficiency* give evidence of left ventricular hypertrophy on the electrocardiogram by the time the patients are symptomatic or in need of surgical correction. Exceptions do occur. *Mitral stenosis* produces increased pressure in the left atrium, causing this chamber to hypertrophy and dilate, and the result is reflected as a broad notched P wave in leads II and III, indicating left atrial enlargement, otherwise called P mitrale. Similar examples can be extended to all other valvular lesions. *Hypertension* acts similarly to aortic stenosis, since it also causes a pressure overload of the left ventricle, producing left ventricular hypertrophy. It should be noted that left ventricular hypertrophy identified by electrocardiogram does not necessarily mean a fixed increase of the muscle mass of the left ventricle, since treating the hypertension will commonly improve the electrocardiogram, and in some cases may cause it to revert to normal.

Arrhythmias. Although an astute examiner can make a specific diagnosis of a rhythm disorder by examining the radial pulse, the venous pulsations, and the quality of the heart sound, the simplest and most accurate method of arrhythmia diagnosis is by electrocardiogram. In selected cases, further investigations by intracardiac electrocardiography (see p. 60) may be necessary before a definite diagnosis can be established. Any deviation of the rhythm from the arbitrarily set sinus rhythm of 60 to 100 is considered to be an arrhythmia; some are trivial and considered to be usual elements of a normal heart, such as sinus arrhythmia or sinus tachycardia.

Extrasystoles. Premature atrial contractions (PACs) can be seen in an otherwise normal heart. If frequent, they may indicate atrial disease and herald the onset of atrial fibrillation. *Premature ventricular contractions (PVCs)* may be considered benign if seen in a healthy young individual without other evidence of cardiac disease. They may herald ventricular tachycardia or fibrillation, especially if seen in a setting of myocardial ischemia, severe heart disease, or acute myocardial infarction, in which the ventricular fibrillatory threshold is lowered. Premature ventricular contractions in the presence of organic heart disease are thought to be malignant if they are multiform, appear in pairs, or are early and appear on the T wave of the preceding complex. This has generally been true in acute myocardial infarction, but the value of this fact in detecting malignant premature ventricular contractions in chronic heart disease remains unclear. Three or more PVCs are commonly designated as ventricular tachycardia. In the presence of organic heart disease, usually coronary artery disease, frequent premature ventricular contractions markedly increase the risk of sudden death; on the other hand, the value of suppressing these premature beats in preventing sudden death is not well established.

Ectopic tachycardia. Atrial fibrillation is the most common of significant atrial arrhythmias. Its presence almost always indicates organic heart disease, usually mitral valve disease or coronary artery disease. Although the diagnosis can be suspected because of an irregularly irregular pulse, an electrocardiogram is essential for an exact diagnosis. Frequent premature beats can mimic the pulse of atrial fibrillation, while a regular pulse may be seen in atrial fibrillation with a high degree of A-V block. This may indicate digitalis excess.

Paroxysmal atrial tachycardia (PAT). This disorder implies functional abnormality of the A-V node and is commonly seen in otherwise healthy, young people free of significant heart disease.

Atrial flutter. This is another common atrial arrhythmia that usually indicates the presence of organic heart disease. It is commonly seen in acute pericarditis.

Ventricular tachycardia. Ventricular tachycardia is rarely seen in an otherwise normal heart, usually indicates severe heart disease, and dictates prompt and accurate diagnosis and treatment. Occasionally the surface electrocardiogram is inadequate in a definitive diagnosis of this disorder because of the difficulty in distinguishing it from a supraventricular tachycardia with aberrant conduction. In such a situation, if permitted by the clinical setting, an intracardiac electrocardiogram can settle the diagnosis.

Ventricular fibrillation. This arrhythmia is the end stage of severe organic heart disease, but it can also be induced by drugs (such as digitalis), electrolyte abnormalities (marked hypokalemia and marked hypomagnesemia), or electrocution. It is thought to be the most common cause of sudden death. This extreme rhythm disorder permits no effective cardiac output. Irreversible brain damage and subsequent death follow if effective resuscitative measures are not instituted in three to five minutes. As a rule, one should not wait to make an electrocardiographic diagnosis of ventricular fibrillation before instituting such measures.

Wolff-Parkinson-White syndrome (WPW). This syndrome has the clinical picture of frequent supraventricular tachycardias with an increased risk of sudden death. The diagnosis is made only by electrocardiography, in which the characteristic features are a short P-R (or P-Q) interval measuring 0.10 seconds or less, widened QRS complexes of 0.11 to 0.14 seconds, and a slurred onset of the QRS complex, commonly known as the delta wave. The QRS complexes resemble those of bundle branch block with associated ST-T abnormalities. In the presence of this disorder, diagnosis of acute myocardial infarction or ventricular hypertrophy may be difficult or impossible to make.

Heart block. Heart block is commonly classified as first degree heart block, which indicates P-R prolongation; second degree heart block, which indicates occasionally nonconducted P waves; and complete or third degree heart block, which indicates nonconducted P waves.

First degree heart block may be secondary to drugs (commonly digitalis), inflammation (myocarditis), or infiltration of the myocardium by a tumor of amyloid. First degree heart block indicates a significant abnormality, but in itself warrants no treatment.

Second degree heart block commonly indicates organic heart disease, but again can be due to metabolic changes or drug toxicity. It is frequently seen in acute myocardial infarction, with type I second degree heart block (progressive prolongation of the P-R interval preceding a nonconducted P wave) accompanying inferior wall infarction and type II second degree heart block (nonconducted P wave preceded and followed by P-R intervals that are all the same length) usually accompanying the anteroseptal myocardial infarction. In the latter, especially, most authorities advocate the use of a prophylactic pacemaker.

Third degree heart block is usually caused by degenerative disease of the conduction system. Coronary artery disease is the second most common cause. This arrhythmia can also be seen in traumatic or inflammatory disease or drug toxicity. Occurring in adults it usually causes significant hemodynamic impairment and can cause syncope (Stokes-Adams syndrome) or death. As a rule, permanent pacing is used in all adult patients. In infants and children, especially in the presence of a stable, narrow ventricular complex and in the absence of symptoms of syncope or dizziness, a pacemaker is not recommended because of the generally favorable course of congenital complete heart block in children as well as the special problems of pacemakers in this age group. A close follow-up of these patients is mandatory.

Bundle branch block is classically viewed as right bundle branch block or left bundle branch block, but in recent years recognition of anterior and posterior branches of the left bundle have been recognized. In the presence of left bundle branch block, diagnosis of myocardial infarction or ventricular hypertrophy may be difficult or impossible to make. Right bundle branch block does not mask a diagnosis of myocardial infarction and may be the clue to silent coronary artery disease. It is commonly seen postoperatively, especially after repair of ventricular septal defects or in the presence of atrial septal defect. Bifascicular block (right bundle branch block and left anterior hemiblock or left posterior hemiblock) in the presence of acute myocardial infarction usually indicates massive myocardial damage with a poor prognosis. Although pacemakers have been used electively (or prophylactically) in these patients, their use is controversial and the salvage rate has been low. In chronic bifascicular block if syncope occurs and is demonstrated to be caused by intermittent second degree or complete heart block, pacemakers are effective in preventing recurrences.

Congenital heart disease. Congenital heart disease in infants, as well as in adults, is commonly accompanied by an abnormal electrocardiogram. The electrocardiogram is characteristic and can lead to an exact diagnosis in a few cases such as endocardial cushion defect, atrial septal defect of the ostium primum type, and transposition of the great vessels with ventricular inversion. More frequently, the abnormality helps in localizing the disease to the right or the left side of the heart. Of course, in infants and children a different set of criteria for normals must be used.

The effects of drugs and electrolytes on the electrocardiogram

Digitalis is commonly used in patients with heart disease and can mimic many of the diagnostic changes of the electrocardiogram. It is important to be familiar with the usual electrocardiographic abnormalities produced by this drug. In normal therapeutic doses digitalis causes sagging of the S-T segment with flattening of the T waves, shortened Q-T interval, and slight prolongation of the P-R interval (Table

Table 4-1. Effect of drugs and electrolytes on the electrocardiogram

Drug or electrolyte	QRS complex	S-T segment	P wave	T wave	U wave	P-R segment	Q-T interval
Digitalis		Sagging		Flattens		Prolongs	Shortens
Quinidine	Widens (toxic)	Depresses	Widens and notches (toxic)	Flattens or inverts			Prolongs
Propranolol				Normal or slightly higher		Prolongs	Shortens
Diphenyl-hydantoin						Shortens	Shortens
Potassium							
Hyperkalemia	Widens	Depresses (>6.5 mEq/l)	Widens (>7.5 mEq/l)	Tall and peaked (5.5-6.5 mEq/l)		Prolongs (>7.5 mEq/l)	
Hypokalemia		Sagging		Notching, then inversion	Prominent		Prolongs (due to U wave)
Calcium							
Hypercalcemia				Widens and rounds			Shortens
Hypocalcemia							Prolongs

4-1). In the presence of atrial fibrillation it also slows the ventricular rate, or it may produce a reversion to normal sinus rhythm. In digitalis excess the following arrhythmias are commonly noted: marked P-R prolongation, second and third degree heart block, and paroxysmal atrial tachycardia with an irregular ventricular response or with block. Digitalis toxicity should be strongly suspected in the presence of ventricular premature beats with bigeminy, multifocal premature beats, pairs of PVCs, or runs of ventricular tachycardia. In the presence of atrial fibrillation, digitalis excess or toxicity may produce a regular pulse due to high degree A-V block and an accelerated junctional focus.

Quinidine produces prolongation of the Q-T interval, with widening and notching of the P waves in therapeutic doses. There could be some S-T segment depression and flattening or inversion of the T waves. When therapeutic levels in the blood are exceeded, the toxic effects noted are varying degrees of A-V block, widening of the QRS complexes over 50% of the normal, and ventricular arrhythmias, including ventricular tachycardia or fibrillation—thus the term "quinidine syncope."

Propranolol (Inderal) predictably slows the sinus rate and produces sinus bradycardia with slight prolongation of the P-R interval. The Q-T interval is shortened and the T waves may remain normal or be slightly higher (Table 4-1). In atrial fibrillation propranolol will slow the ventricular response.

Diphenylhydantoin (Dilantin) is used in the treatment of digitalis toxicity. It tends to shorten the P-R interval and the Q-T interval without having a significant effect on the QRS complex (Table 4-1). This characteristic of diphenylhydantoin is considered to make it the drug of choice in the treatment of digitalis toxicity in the presence of prolongation of the P-R segment or first or second degree heart block.

The effect of lidocaine on the electrocardiogram is minor. Some studies have shown increased intraventricular conduction delay, while other studies have refuted this. For practical purposes no significant change on the surface electrocardiogram is recorded.

The electrocardiogram is most useful in diagnosing and following the progression of hyperkalemia and the effect of therapy. The first electrocardiographic manifestation of hyperkalemia occurs with blood concentrations in the range of 5.5 to 6.5 mEq/l. At this level the T waves become characteristically tall and peaked. With further elevations in the plasma potassium concentration, there is a decreased amplitude of the R waves with increased S waves, S-T depressions, and prolongation of the QRS duration and the P-R interval. When the plasma potassium concentration exceeds 7.5 mEq/l, intra-atrial conduction disturbances develop and are reflected in broad low amplitude P waves and P-R interval prolongation (Table 4-1). At higher potassium levels, the P wave disappears altogether, and the QRS becomes markedly widened and moves into a smooth diphasic (sine) wave. The final stage, if untreated, is ventricular tachycardia, flutter, fibrillation, and standstill.

In hypokalemia there is initially an apparent prolongation of the Q-T interval. This is caused by the appearance of a U wave that merges with the T wave and may cause notching of the T wave. T wave inversion follows and then sagging of the S-T segment. The administration of potassium rapidly reverses these changes.

Hypercalcemia characteristically shortens the S-T segment of the Q-T interval and may also widen and cause a rounding of the T waves. Hypocalcemia causes a prolongation of the Q-T interval (Table 4-1).

Important points to remember

A normal electrocardiogram does not rule out severe organic heart disease. This fact may seem to be obvious on the surface, but it is frequently disregarded. Severe obstructive disease of all major coronary arteries without myocardial infarction or active ischemia of the heart is a common situation that could produce a perfectly normal electrocardiogram.

A definitely abnormal electrocardiogram does not necessarily signify heart disease. As discussed, S-T abnormalities, even pronounced, can be due to CNS lesions or be produced by drugs, electrolytes, or other causes.

Electrocardiographic interpretations should be made in the context of the clinical situation. Serious errors will be made if the clinical data are not used in interpreting an electrocardiogram.

The limitations of the standard resting electrocardiogram should be recognized. It is at most a one minute record of the heart's electrical activity and it is recorded at rest, without stressing the heart. Whenever necessary further tests should be used, such as the Holter monitor for arrhythmia diagnosis or stress electrocardiography for diagnosis of coronary artery disease. These will be discussed in the following sections.

Ambulatory electrocardiography (Holter monitoring)

Ambulatory electrocardiography is an extension of the resting electrocardiogram and, as commonly used, records one lead. However, some newer models have the capability for two-lead recording.

The electrocardiogram is recorded on magnetic tape, reels, or cassettes in portable recorders that can be worn on the patient's belt or shoulder and record the electrocardiogram continuously for twelve or twenty-four hours in essentially unrestricted activity. The tapes are scanned rapidly by electrocardioscanners, and abnormalities or selected areas of interest are printed out in real time. Recently, computers have been utilized in the rapid processing of tapes and have vastly expanded the ability to process a large number of tapes.

Clinical value

The clinical uses or values of ambulatory electrocardiography are many. Obviously, it enables a much larger sample of the electrocardiogram to be recorded; instead of 60 to 100 complexes noted on the usual resting electrocardiogram, this samples 50 to 100 thousand beats on a 10- to 24-hour record. A second value is that it includes the electrocardiogram during rest, during usual unrestricted activity, as well as during sleep. Many abnormalities of the electrocardiogram that have in the past gone undetected during the patient's sleep are now being recognized.

Indications for the use of ambulatory monitoring

1. *Diagnosis of arrhythmias.* In patients complaining of dizziness or palpitations or actually having episodes of syncope, the ambulatory electrocardiogram is an invaluable diagnostic tool. If the rhythm disorder *and* the symptoms are shown to be coincident, then an exact diagnosis of an elusive disorder can be made.
2. *Monitoring of high risk patients.* Holter monitoring is especially useful when the patient is discharged from the hospital soon after a myocardial infarction.
3. *Evaluation of the effectiveness of drug treatment of arrhythmias.*
4. *Diagnosis of ischemic heart disease.* Not uncommonly, ischemic S-T depressions can be noted on the ambulatory electrocardiogram during periods of stress, be it exertion, emotional stress, heavy meals, or cigarette smoking. Sometimes ischemic changes are recorded during the patient's sleep; these are commonly associated with periods of rapid eye movement sleep with dreams, associated sinus tachycardia, and possibly a rise in the blood pressure.

Prinzmetal's angina manifests S-T elevation in the presence of angina and is associated with proximal high grade coronary artery obstructive lesions. The exercise electrocardiogram may be negative and show no ischemic S-T changes or pain. In such a case the ambulatory electrocardiogram can be very useful in detecting the S-T abnormalities that may occur during rest.

Contraindications and limitations

There are no absolute or relative contraindications for ambulatory electrocardiography; however, the limitations are several. It is a costly procedure, ranging from $100 to $200 for a 10- to 24-hour tape, recording, and analysis. Further use of computerization may overcome this hurdle. Another limitation is availability; but as the value of ambulatory electrocardiography becomes more widely recognized, it will be available on a larger scale. The commonly used one-lead system limits the diagnostic usefulness, especially if the search is for S-T depressions. But as newer systems increase the number of recording leads available, this limitation also will be overcome.

Ambulatory electrocardiography is an invaluable extension of the resting electrocardiogram and should be a part of any complete cardiac laboratory. It remains a totally noninvasive method, free of risks except that of misdiagnosis (inability to recognize artifacts) and overdiagnosis (detection of benign arrhythmias) with the subsequent risk of unnecessary treatment.

Exercise electrocardiography

The exercise electrocardiogram was initially a twelve-lead electrocardiogram performed after the patient had stepped up and down a set of stairs of a standard height a certain number of times. Again, like the electrocardiogram, the basic concept has remained unchanged since it was popularized by Arthur Master in 1929, but advances in electronics and gadgetry have produced new equipment. In its basic form, the test consists of a gradually increasing level of exercise while the electrocardiogram is being monitored. All twelve leads can be monitored. The entire recording can be stored on a magnetic tape and subsequently analyzed, or recordings can be obtained intermittently. Newer models incorporate automatic rate meter and S-T segment analyzing computers. Various investigators have proposed different protocols for the gradually increasing work load, and the most widely used is that proposed by Robert Bruce. From the five to ten minutes of the exercise electrocardiogram recorded in such a standardized manner, a large amount of valuable information is obtained, which includes: (1) the minutes of exercise—given a standard load, the maximum oxygen consumption can be derived; (2) the heart rate achieved at the peak of exercise—if blood pressure is obtained at the same time, a heart rate × blood pressure "double product" is obtained that is a good approximation of myocardial or heart work; (3) the degree of S-T depression that relates to myocardial ischemia; and (4) arrhythmias provoked during exercise or more often during early recovery.

Clinical value

The values of exercise electrocardiography are many. In coronary artery disease, the resting electrocardiogram, when there is no myocardial infarction, is frequently normal, or the changes are nonspecific. In this situation the stress electrocardiogram is commonly abnormal and frequently quite diagnostic, by indicating flat or down-sloping ischemic S-T depression.

Like many other tests in medicine, this one has its limitations. False negative tests, even when a maximum heart rate is achieved, may be seen in as many as 25% of patients with coronary artery disease. Massive coronary occlusion with myocardial infarction can be seen in patients with normal maximal exercise electrocardiograms performed days or weeks prior to the insult.

There can also be false positive tests, that is, "ischemic" S-T depression in the absence of coronary artery disease. Causes for this could be digitalis administration, electrolyte abnormalities, or no cause may be found. It is possible that some people with a "false positive" test may be suffering from disease of small vessels in the heart, currently not visualized by coronary angiographic techniques. This concept is presently under intensive investigation.

Another value of treadmill testing is in diagnosis of arrhythmias. Although ambulatory monitoring remains the method of choice in detecting suspected arrhythmias, the ease of performing exercise electrocardiography has caused more interest to be shown in its use for this purpose. This is especially the case if the arrhythmias are suspected to occur during exercise, and to be major arrhythmias of a life-threatening nature. In such patients one is reluctant to advise ambulatory monitoring during exercise; however, these arrhythmias could be provoked during an exercise electrocardiogram in a controlled setting with facilities for immediate treatment.

This test is also a useful adjunct in the evaluation of the patient's functional capacity or "physical fitness." It is useful in evaluating methods of therapy, including drugs or surgery, such as coronary artery bypass surgery, as well as in obtaining an objective evaluation of the patient's disability in situations where a history is confusing or difficult to obtain. The exercise ECG is useful in exercise prescription for the rehabilitation of patients following myocardial infarction or cardiac surgery.

Limitations

The major limitation of stress electrocardiography is the high, and for some people unacceptable, level of false positive and false negative results in attempts to diagnose ischemic heart disease. A second limitation is cost, which is between that of a resting electrocardiogram and a ten-hour ambulatory electrocardiogram.

Indications

The indications for stress electrocardiography are many. Like the resting electrocardiogram, it can be considered an extension of the physical examination. Specific indications were discussed in the section on the value of the test.

Contraindications

This test, unlike the resting electrocardiogram, does have some contraindications. Among these are any severe acute illnesses, specifically acute myocardial infarction, myocarditis, or severe arrhythmias. Other contraindications would be uncompensated congestive heart failure and drug toxicity.

Pitfalls

In stress electrocardiography, confusion can arise in diagnosing ischemic S-T depression. Junctional S-T depression, which is not flat or downsloping of 1 mm or more, can be misdiagnosed as positive for ischemia. As already mentioned, digitalis can produce or accentuate ischemic S-T changes as can electrolyte abnormalities, specifically hypokalemia.

Nitroglycerin enables the patient with coronary artery disease to perform a higher level of exercise and possibly produce less arrhythmias. Thus, a patient's drug history immediately prior to testing should be noted.

If careful attention is not given to details of the testing and the patient uses the handrail for support, standardization of the test will be ruined and conclusions can be erroneous.

Another pitfall is that patients do learn how to perform the test and very commonly perform better on a second test, compared with a first test, without any intervention. Usually this learning does not progress from a second to third test and so on.

Risks

Risks include mortality of one in 10,000 tests performed, which is usually from ventricular fibrillation that was not successfully resuscitated. Complications necessitating hospitalization are in the range of 0.2% and include myocardial infarction, prolonged bouts of chest pain, severe arrhythmias, or hypertensive episodes. These risks can be minimized by screening patients by means of a history and physical examination, a resting electrocardiogram prior to testing, and availability and familiarity with resuscitative equipment.

Informed consent is not necessary for this test, but is preferred by many centers.

Vectorcardiography (VCG)

The vectorcardiogram (VCG) was introduced by Frank Wilson in 1938. Whereas the ECG displays local electrical forces of the heart at a given time and point, the vectorcardiogram displays the balance of these forces at any instant. It is a plot of voltage against voltage in three-dimensional space and is a useful addition to the scalar ECG, reinforcing and making the understanding of scalar electrocardiography more complete.

Clinical value

The diagnostic advantages of the VCG over the ECG are as follows:
1. In determining the cause of slowing of electrical waveforms; specifically, it is helpful in the diagnosis of the initial slowing of W-P-W syndrome (Wolff-Parkinson-White syndrome) and the differentiation of the bundle branch blocks from other causes of widened QRS complexes
2. In establishing the differential diagnosis between inferior wall myocardial infarction and left anterior hemiblock when there are S waves with embryonic r waves in leads II, III, and aV_F

3. In the differential diagnosis of RBBB from right ventricular hypertrophy
4. In detecting left ventricular hypertrophy in the presence of LBBB; analysis of the vector angle and magnitude can be helpful
5. As an adjunct to scalar electrocardiography, increasing the diagnostic yield by approximately 10%
6. In the differential diagnosis of right ventricular hypertrophy versus true posterior myocardial infarction, helping to determine if the ECG pattern is due to either a loss of posterior forces (true posterior M.I.) or a gain of anterior forces (right ventricular hypertrophy)

   Although the vectorcardiogram at present has not gained as wide an acceptance or use as the scalar electrocardiogram in most community hospitals, recent introduction of computerized techniques in obtaining and interpreting vectorcardiograms will undoubtedly help in popularizing this diagnostic tool.

Routine radiographic examination of the heart

The chest x-ray examination in two projections, posterior-anterior (PA) and lateral, provides valuable information about the size and contour of the heart. Anatomic changes of individual chambers are seen in the right and left anterior oblique projections. These projections are illustrated in Figs. 4-3 to 4-6. Before the advent of echocardiography, radiographic examination was the simplest, most accurate way of assessing cardiac size, a fact that has made percussion of the chest for heart size in the physical examination of the patient almost a lost art.

Clinical value

The simplest and most frequently used measurement is the cardiothoracic ratio. This measurement is achieved by adding the longest distance from the midline of

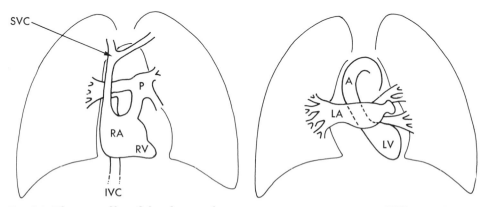

Fig. 4-3. The x-ray film of the chest in the posterior-anterior projection. SVC, superior vena cava; IVC, inferior vena cava; RA, right atrium; RV, right ventricle; P, pulmonary artery; LA, left atrium; LV, left ventricle; A, aorta.

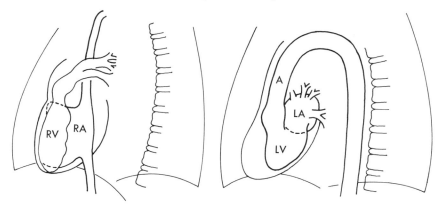

Fig. 4-4. The x-ray film of the chest in the left lateral projection.

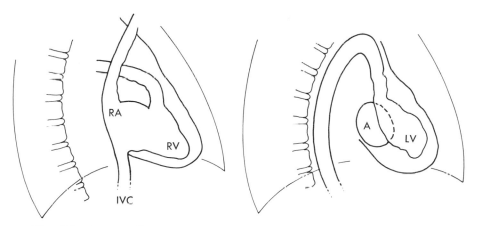

Fig. 4-5. The x-ray film of the chest in the right anterior oblique projection.

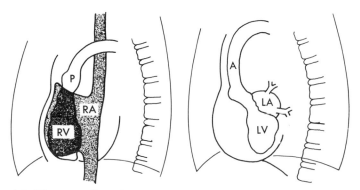

Fig. 4-6. The x-ray film of the chest in the left anterior oblique projection.

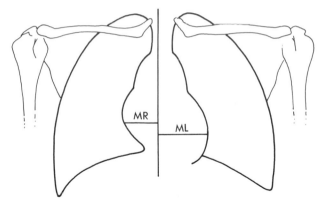

Fig. 4-7. The cardiothoracic ratio derived by adding the midright (MR) and midleft (ML) measurements. The sum is then divided by the longest transverse diameter of the chest.

the chest to the right and left sides of the heart (Fig. 4-7). The transverse diameter of the heart equals the sum of the longest mid-to-right and the longest mid-to-left measurements from a line drawn in the midline of the chest. This transverse diameter is divided by the longest transverse diameter of the chest, arriving at a cardiothoracic ratio. This is a relatively crude way of assessing cardiac size, but because it is easily obtained, it is commonly used. Generally a cardiothoracic ratio over 50% is considered cardiac enlargement. Some reasonable assessment of individual chamber enlargement can be made from inspection of the plain chest film in the PA and lateral projections.

Inspection of the lung fields. Overcirculation or undercirculation of the lung fields as compared with normal circulation is most helpful in the differential diagnosis of congenital heart diseases. In the presence of a left-to-right shunt there are signs of increased circulation in the pulmonary vessels; in the presence of a right-to-left shunt there is evidence of undercirculation. Patterns of pulmonary veins, their size and prominence, as well as the presence or absence of pulmonary lymphatic markings help in the diagnosis of elevated pulmonary venous pressure, which is a common sign of congestive heart failure.

Pulmonary edema can be of two kinds, alveolar and interstitial. Alveolar edema is characteristic of acute left-sided heart failure and is manifested by bilateral confluent densities that start centrally and spread peripherally, commonly referred to as the butterfly-wing pattern. In interstitial edema, fluid accumulates in the interstitial tissues of the lungs and produces a generalized haziness and clouding of the vascular shadows. When such fluid collects in the interlobular septa of the lung, septal lines are formed that are referred to as Kerley's lines.

Inspection of the pleural spaces. Approximately 250 ml of pleural effusion is necessary for an accurate radiologic diagnosis. This is usually manifested as blunting of the costophrenic angle. Larger effusions can also accumulate, approximately a liter, and may be an accompaniment of congestive heart failure or be independent of heart disease and indicate the presence of lung disease. Diagnosis of pleural effusion is

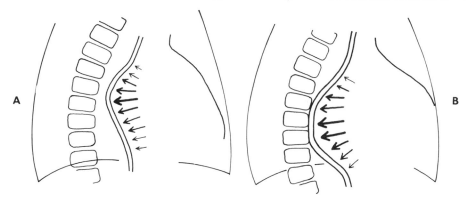

Fig. 4-8. The x-ray film of the chest obtained after the patient has swallowed barium (a "cardiac series"). Note the moderate, **A**, and marked, **B**, degrees of left atrial enlargement reflected in the displacement of the atrium by the barium-filled esophagus. This is a right anterior oblique projection.

discussed on p. 99. Occasionally, pleural effusions are hidden under the lung (subpulmonic effusion) and therefore do not obliterate the costophrenic angle. These effusions can be detected by obtaining the film with the patient in the lateral position, commonly referred to as the lateral decubitus film.

Inspection of the rib cage. Inspection may provide a clue for coarctation of the aorta where collateral circulation from enlarged intercostal arteries would produce characteristic deformity or notching of the rib margins.

Cardiac series. The ability to make a more accurate diagnosis of specific chamber enlargement is enhanced by obtaining a cardiac series, in which a bolus of barium is swallowed by the patient, opacifying the posterior-lying esophagus. In addition to the PA and lateral films two oblique films are obtained. In the cardiac series an enlarged left atrium or even an enlarged aorta could be noted displacing the barium-filled esophagus (Fig. 4-8). This, along with the additional projections, would aid in the diagnosis of left or right ventricular enlargement.

CO_2 injection and cardiac fluoroscopy. Carbon dioxide (CO_2) may be injected into a peripheral vein for the diagnosis of pericardial effusion. After a brief period, x-ray films are taken with the patient in the left lateral position. The carbon dioxide acts as a contrast material within the right atrial chamber, defining the thickness of the right atrial and pericardial wall. At present this technique is not commonly used and is being replaced by the echocardiogram because of its diagnostic simplicity and accuracy.

Cardiac fluoroscopy is most useful in detecting calcifications of various parts of the heart. Introduction of image intensifiers has decreased the overall radiation hazard of this test and has improved the quality of the images seen. Cardiac fluoroscopy is useful in detecting calcification in the coronary artery system. Although the diagnostic method of choice for detection and semiquantitation of coronary artery disease is by selective coronary angiography (see p. 88), cardiac fluoroscopy is a useful screening tool for this purpose. Approximately 75% of the patients with coronary artery disease have calcification of their coronary artery system, but 20% of the patients (especially older patients) with normal coronary angiograms also reveal calcification of the coronary arteries. Calcification of the various valves of the heart, specifically the aortic and the mitral valves, is unequivocal evidence of disease of these valves. Although heavier calcification correlates with more significant disease of the valves (usually narrowing), an exact correlation cannot be made. Other cardiac diseases in which calcification is helpful in the diagnosis are tumors of the heart, calcification of the pericardium in constrictive pericarditis, and calcification of the myocardium secondary to old myocardial infarction.

Limitations

The chest x-ray examination of the heart can be perfectly normal in the presence of severe organic disease of the heart. The information revealed is mainly of a static nature, with the dynamic aspects of the working heart not detected.

Variations of heart size in systole as compared with diastole also diminish the accuracy of detection of cardiac enlargement.

Indications

The chest x-ray examination and cardiac series are used almost as an extension of the physical examination and are performed on patients with all kinds of cardiac disease as well as in screening of the normal population. As discussed, cardiac fluoroscopy is indicated in situations where there is suspicion of calcification of various parts of the heart.

Contraindications

There is no absolute contraindication, since the risk is limited to a mimimal exposure to ionizing radiation, a risk that increases with exposure. This becomes more important in young children and in pregnant women in whom studies should be performed only when necessary and the gonads or the fetus should routinely be shielded.

Pitfalls

In the use of radiographic examination of the heart, diagnostic errors can originate either from the recording technique or during the interpretation of the information.

Technical errors. Films exposed during expiration may produce a false impression of an enlarged heart and pulmonary vascular congestion. This also becomes exaggerated in the patient who is obese with a high diaphragm and enlarged pericardial fat. Overpenetration may produce disappearance of pulmonary vascular markings. Rotation of the patient may produce a false appearance of enlargement or may produce magnification of various vessels.

Errors of interpretation. In the presence of a pectus excavatum deformity of the chest, the heart may be displaced posteriorly and produce a false impression of cardiomegaly. In pectus carinatum deformity of the chest, the anterior-posterior diameter is increased and possible enlargement of the right ventricle may go undetected. Patients with a straight dorsal spine may simulate cardiomegaly, especially on the lateral projection. In patients with severe kyphoscoliosis, accurate assessment of cardiac size and pulmonary vasculature may be impossible. A portable chest x-ray examination cannot be used to assess cardiac size, although it can be helpful in assessing the degree of pulmonary congestion.

Further pitfalls in the interpretation of x-ray films of the chest are many, but discussion of them would be beyond the scope of this book.

Use of blood tests in cardiac disease

A multitude of blood tests are used in evaluation of the cardiac patient. Like the electrocardiogram and the chest x ray, they are an extension of the physical examination and constitute an integral part of a complete evaluation. Recent automation has further popularized these tests by making them easily available and also reducing the cost.

Cardiac enzymes

These have been discussed in Chapter 1 and are briefly mentioned here. Normal blood levels for these enzymes as well as the organs in which the content is high can be found in Fig. 4-9 and Table 4-2.

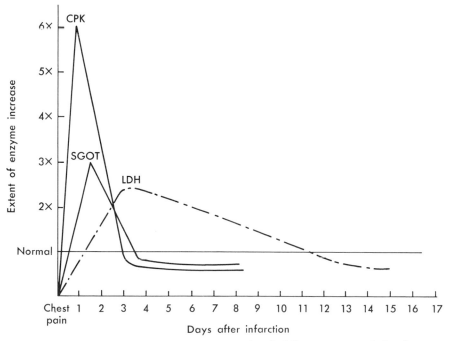

Fig. 4-9. Typical changes in serum enzyme levels following myocardial infarction.

Table 4-2. Normal blood levels and enzyme distribution in cells*

Enzyme	*Tissue*	*Normal blood levels*
Creatine phosphokinase (CPK)	Heart Brain Skeletal muscle	Female 5-25 U/ml Male 5-35 U/ml Female 55-170 U/l at 37° C Male 30-135 U/l at 37° C
Serum glutamic oxalacetic transaminase (SGOT)	Heart Kidney Red cells Brain Pancreas Lung Liver Skeletal muscle	10-40 Karmen units 6-18 IU/l
Lactic dehydrogenase (LDH)	Heart Kidney Red cells Brain Lymph nodes Spleen Leukocytes Pancreas Lung Liver Skeletal muscle	80-120 Wacker units 150-450 Wrobleski unit 71-207 IU/l

*The normal levels vary from laboratory to laboratory according to the test used.

SGOT (serum glutamic oxalic transaminase). Levels of this enzyme begin to rise in about eight hours, peak in twenty-four to forty-eight hours (Fig. 4-9), and return to normal in four to eight days following a myocardial infarction. Damage to other tissues besides the heart may elevate this enzyme and cause a false diagnosis of myocardial infarction.

LDH (lactic dehydrogenase). Elevated LDH levels usually persist longer than SGOT levels and can be helpful if the patient is seen several days after the onset of myocardial infarction (Fig. 4-9).

CPK (creatine phosphokinase). This enzyme is found in the heart as well as in skeletal muscle and the brain, but is not elevated appreciably in damage to red blood cells or the liver. There are many causes for elevated CPK, including vigorous exercise, skeletal muscle disease, intramuscular injections, cerebral infarctions, and myocardial infarction. People with an unusually large muscle mass, such as athletes, have a higher CPK value than the general population. CPK is separated into three isoenzymes, labeled as CPK-MM, CPK-BB, and CPK-MB. The myocardium contains MB fraction as well as some MM fraction. In myocardial injury the elevated fraction is of the MB type. In skeletal muscle injury, CPK elevation is of the MM activity. Recently,

Table 4-3. Concentrations of C, TG, or LDL which, if exceeded, clearly indicate hyperlipidemia

Age	C*	TG*	LDL*
>29 years	240	140	170
30-39 years	270	150	190
40-49 years	310	160	190
50+	330	190	210

*C = Cholesterol; TG = Triglyceride; LDL = Low density lipoproteins
Reproduced with permission from Frederickson, D. S.: A physician's guide to hyperlipidemia, Mod. Concepts Cardiovasc. Dis. 41(7), 1972, American Heart Association, Inc.

attempts have been made to quantitate the total CPK rise, to relate this to the amount of muscle necrosis in myocardial infarction, and, in turn, to relate this to the prognosis of the patient. In general the larger the CPK rise, the larger the infarct area and the poorer the prognosis for the patient.

Clinical value. At present the value of these enzymes in diagnosis of myocardial infarction is: (1) as an adjunct to the history, physical examination, and the ECG in confirming the clinical impression of myocardial infarction and (2) in following the course of the myocardial infarction and especially in detecting extension of myocardial infarction where the electrocardiogram may not change.

Blood lipids

Elevated blood lipid as an abnormality in relation to coronary artery disease has received much attention recently. The blood lipids (cholesterol, triglycerides, and phospholipids) circulate in the plasma bound to protein, thus the term "lipoproteins." Electrophoresis is the method used to separate the lipoproteins, and from this several classifications have evolved. For practical purposes two types of hyperlipidemia are important in cardiac disease: type 2, in which the cholesterol is elevated and the triglycerides are normal or mildly elevated, and type 4, in which the cholesterol is normal and the triglycerides are elevated.

The normal designation for cholesterol and triglycerides, as discussed in Chapter 1, varies among populations and age groups (Table 4-3). The generally accepted upper limit of normal is 250 mg for cholesterol and 150 mg for triglycerides.

The association of hyperlipidemia and coronary artery disease is well established, an association that is more striking in the younger population. Although there is no conclusive proof at this time that lowering abnormally elevated lipids will hold or retard the progression of coronary artery disease, it is prudent to detect these elevations and to use dietary and, if indicated, drug measures to bring these levels to within normal range or at least to lower levels. It is generally agreed that the lower the blood lipids, the less chance for acquiring coronary artery disease.

There are two common pitfalls in the measurement of blood lipids: the patient has to be fasting if useful information is to be obtained, and there can be marked fluctuations in the same patient in day-to-day measurements. Therefore, besides fasting, the patient should have several measurements before a definite diagnosis of hyperlipidemia is made and dietary and/or drug therapy is instituted.

Blood glucose and glucose tolerance test (GTT)

An abnormal glucose tolerance test is commonly associated with hyperlipidemia and obesity, and is an additional risk factor for coronary artery disease. Fasting blood glucose measurements will detect the overt symptomatic diabetic patient. The value of the glucose tolerance test in detecting the asymptomatic patient with diabetes lies in defining this risk factor. Generally, no treatment is necessary except weight reduction in the obese.

Pitfalls. Two pitfalls in the measurement of the glucose tolerance test are: (1) the patient should not have a below-average carbohydrate intake before the test and (2) this test should not be done too soon, days to weeks, after a myocardial infarction, since it will often be abnormally elevated.

Other blood tests

Among the other blood tests commonly employed are determinations of electrolytes, blood urea nitrogen (BUN), and serum creatinine. For a complete discussion of these tests refer to Chapter 1.

Abnormalities of electrolytes are common in patients with heart disease and are either secondary to congestive heart failure or in combination with side effects to drug therapy for this condition.

Chronic congestive heart failure causes total body, as well as myocardial, potassium and magnesium depletion and in severe stages, when water is not restricted, may also produce lowering of the serum sodium level (hyponatremia). Diuretics used to decrease total body sodium may also produce hyponatremia if water is not restricted. They commonly produce total body potassium depletion and this *may* be detected as a lowering of the serum potassium (hypokalemia), although significant total body potassium depletion can occur in the absence of hypokalemia.

Creatinine clearance may fall and blood urea nitrogen level may rise in severe congestive heart failure.

Measurement of drug levels in plasma

Monitoring of blood levels of various cardiac drugs is essential for successful and safe treatment. Of the commonly used drugs, assays for plasma levels are presently available for digoxin, quinidine, procainamide, diphenylhydantoin, lidocaine, and propranolol. The therapeutic and toxic blood levels for these drugs is displayed in Table 4-4.

Miscellaneous blood tests

The complete blood count (CBC) is useful in detection of anemias, which may (1) present as angina in the patient with coronary artery disease, (2) aggravate con-

Table 4-4. Therapeutic and toxic blood levels for cardiac drugs

	Therapeutic blood level	*Toxic blood level*
Digitoxin	14 to 30 ng/ml	Over 30 ng/ml
Digoxin	1.0 to 2.0 ng/ml	Over 3 ng/ml
Propranolol (Inderal)	20 to 50 ng/ml	Over 50 ng/ml
Procainamide (Pronestyl)	4 to 8 mcg/ml	Over 8 mcg/ml
Diphenylhydantoin (Dilantin)	10 to 18 mcg/ml	Over 18 mcg/ml
Quinidine	2.5 to 5 mcg/ml	Over 5 mcg/ml
Lidocaine	1.4 to 6 mcg/ml	Over 6 mcg/ml

gestive heart failure, (3) give a diagnostic clue in subacute bacterial endocarditis, or (4) present evidence of hemolysis in patients with prosthetic valves.

The white blood cell count (WBC) is elevated in patients with myocardial infarction, bacterial endocarditis, and the postmyocardial infarction Dressler syndrome.

The sedimentation rate is elevated in acute myocardial infarction, bacterial endocarditis, Dressler's syndrome and in many other diseases that cause inflammation. It is considered to be characteristically low in congestive heart failure.

The C reactive protein is usually absent in normal people and is elevated in persons with acute rheumatic fever.

Antistreptolysin-O (ASO) titer is elevated after streptococcal infections and can be the clue to diagnosis of acute rheumatic fever.

The VDRL, discussed on p. 178, can be the clue to syphilitic heart disease, usually presenting as aortic insufficiency or disease of the ostia of the coronary arteries.

Prothrombin time is used in initiating and maintaining anticoagulation with oral anticoagulants (drugs such as coumadin). Usually the prothrombin time is kept within 2 to 2.5 times the normal, and that is generally comparable to 20% to 30% of the activity of normal. The partial thromboplastin time (PTT) and the clotting time are used in following patients receiving heparin, and 2 to 2.5 times the normal is the therapeutic range.

Anticoagulation with heparin, and subsequently with Coumadin-type drugs, is used in pulmonary embolism, deep venous thrombosis, cerebral embolism and acute peripheral arterial embolism and is felt to be beneficial in patients with acute myocardial infarction with congestive heart failure during the period of bed rest. Because multiple drugs interfere with the metabolism and reaction of the Coumadin-type anticoagulants, frequent measurements of the prothrombin time and careful checks of the interaction of other drugs are important in minimizing the risk of hemorrhage in patients receiving anticoagulant drugs.

Blood cultures are crucial in the diagnosis of infective endocarditis. It is important to obtain an adequate number of cultures. Generally six cultures are considered adequate. These should be obtained by sterile technique, preferably inoculated at the bedside, and cultured on aerobic, anaerobic, and microaerophilic media.

The common pitfalls in the diagnosis of endocarditis from blood cultures are (1) contamination with a false positive diagnosis and (2) the presence of antibiotics in the patient's serum or possibly the patient being partially treated with antibiotics and having, therefore, false negative cultures.

Arterial blood gas determinations are discussed on p. 98. Patients with myocardial infarction or congestive heart failure commonly manifest abnormalities of the arterial blood gases. Patients who have hypoxemia or desaturation secondary to altered ventilation perfusion ratios usually benefit from oxygen administration in an attempt to keep their saturation 90% or higher. Patients who have myocardial infarctions, especially with pulmonary congestion or edema, commonly hyperventilate, with subsequent lowering of the PCO_2 and mild respiratory alkalosis. In the presence of severe pulmonary edema, hypoventilation with elevation of the PCO_2 and mild respiratory acidosis may occur.

Some drugs used in the treatment of myocardial infarction, especially morphine, produce a predictable drop in the rate and depth of respiration and may, in excessive doses, precipitate hypoventilation with respiratory acidosis. Therefore, in patients who are receiving larger than usual doses of morphine or morphine along with other suppressants, arterial blood gas determinations are indicated to detect and/or avoid respiratory depression.

Carbon monoxide level is elevated in moderate to heavy smokers, as well as in areas of heavy industrial pollution, and may precipitate or exacerbate angina pectoris in the presence of coronary artery disease. Measurement of carbon monoxide levels in the blood can be helpful in detecting unusually heavy industrial exposure as well as the heavy cigarette smoker with angina pectoris.

Urine examination

Measurement of the volume of urine through twenty-four hours is helpful, since in heart failure the night volume may be from 30% to 50% more than the day volume; such nighttime elevation is referred to as nocturia.

The presence of red cells in the urine may be the clue to evidence of infective endocarditis or embolic disease of the kidneys.

Mild proteinuria, 1 to 2 grams per day, can be seen in congestive heart failure. Patients with marked elevation of venous pressure, constrictive pericarditis, or tricuspid insufficiency may present with massive proteinuria, and even with the nephrotic syndrome.

Recently the detection of myoglobin in the urine (myoglobinuria) has been found useful as a sensitive test in the diagnosis of myocardial infarction, but clinical experience with this test remains very limited.

NONINVASIVE SPECIALIZED DIAGNOSTIC METHODS IN CARDIOLOGY

The following is a discussion of the more important tests used in the physician's office and hospital practice of cardiology. These tests are grouped together because they are noninvasive; that is, they do not break the patient's skin or interfere with or alter the events that are being observed. They also pose no risk or significant discomfort to the patient and can be repeated at frequent intervals with absolute safety. There has been increasing interest in these tests, and although presently they do not, with rare exceptions, produce the detailed and accurate information obtained by invasive (such as cardiac catheterization) tests, they complement them in many cases and may soon approach the accuracy of the invasive tests. Tests with proven clinical value are discussed in the order of their general importance or usefulness.

Echocardiography

Echocardiography (ultrasound cardiography) is a relatively recent tool in cardiology and is finding widespread acceptance and use. Stated simply, it is a technique in which echos (reflected ultrasound) from pulsed high frequency sound waves are used to locate and study the movements and the dimensions of various cardiac structures. This is done without the use of injected contrast media. The technique yields direct recordings of the motion of the mitral, aortic, and, with some experience, the tricuspid and the pulmonic valve leaflets, the interventricular septum, and the right and left ventricular walls. It provides accurate measurement of the size of the cardiac cham-

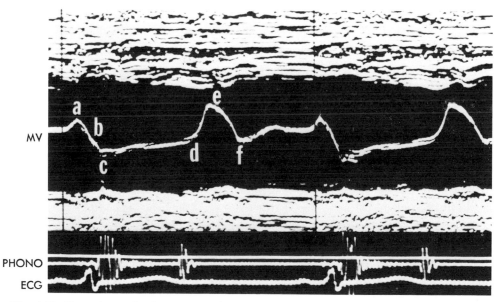

Fig. 4-10. Normal mitral valve. A normal mitral valve trace (MV) has been labeled to identify physiologic events. Atrial systole is followed by a peak (a). Onset of ventricular systole (b) culminates in valve closure (c). A gradual anterior motion occurs during systole. Valve opening starts at point (d) and the valve is fully opened at (e). Posterior movement in diastole (e-f) is an indication of the rate of left atrial emptying. PHONO, Phonocardiogram; ECG, electrocardiogram. (From King, D. L., editor: Diagnostic ultrasound, St. Louis, 1974, The C. V. Mosby Co.)

bers and the changes of these dimensions during the cardiac cycle. It also permits recognition of abnormal filling defects, as in atrial tumors.

Because the ultrasound beam tracks the motion of various cardiac structures over a period of time, it provides a time-motion study of the heart. This technique has given cardiologists the unique opportunity to visualize internal structures of the heart in a totally noninvasive manner and with a degree of sensitivity exceeding that of ordinary x-ray films. The test is usually performed in the echocardiographic laboratory with the patient supine. The transducer (the source of ultrasound as well as the receiver of the reflected ultrasound) is placed on the surface of the chest along the left sternal border, third to fifth interspace, to avoid interference from the lung, as ultrasound transmits very poorly in air.

In acutely ill patients or others who may not be able to be transferred to the echocardiographic laboratory, portable echocardiographic equipment can be used and the complete test performed at the bedside. The echocardiogram is recorded on photographic paper (strip chart recording) or on film (Polaroid). A normal echocardiogram showing mainly the excursions of the mitral value leaflets is shown in Fig. 4-10.

Clinical value

The echocardiogram was first employed as an aid in the diagnosis of mitral stenosis. Fig. 4-11 illustrates the abnormal movement of the mitral valve in a patient with mitral stenosis. In the past eight to ten years echocardiographic application has expanded very rapidly and, as a new tool, its indications are being continuously revised and extended. It is expected that in many of the disorders in which echocardiography now has adjunctive value it will later be of diagnostic value and that it will become useful in additional disorders.

Echocardiography is helpful in the diagnosis of the following disorders: mitral stenosis, tricuspid stenosis, pericardial effusion, atrial septal defects, prolapsing mitral leaflet syndrome, hypertrophic cardiomyopathy (obstructive or nonobstructive), atrial tumors, and multiple congenital defects in neonates and infants. It is also useful in the evaluation of aortic and pulmonic valves for stenosis or insufficiency and mitral insufficiency as well as for assessment of the function of the left ventricle (cardiac output and ejection fraction). In the large group of disorders under coronary artery disease the echocardiogram has been useful in evaluating abnormal left ventricular function secondary to coronary artery disease or myocardial infarction. Presently the echocardiogram is of no value in the diagnosis and evaluation of obstructive disease of the coronary arteries.

Limitations of echocardiography

Although echocardiography is an exciting and fascinating field, it has its limitations. At the present time in approximately 10% to 15% of patients, adequate quality for diagnostic purposes cannot be obtained, due to technical reasons. Because it is a new method, technicians proficient in the performance of the test, as well as physi-

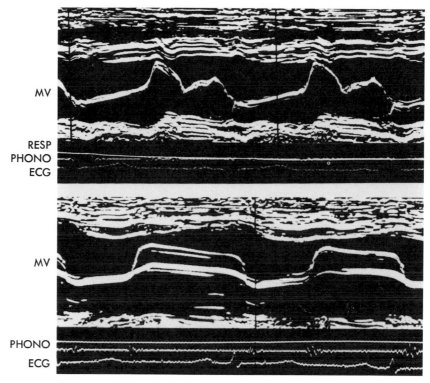

MV

RESP
PHONO
ECG

MV

PHONO
ECG

Fig. 4-11. Mitral stenosis. The upper panel is from a normal subject and shows a sharply peaked early diastolic trace, moderate sized A waves and a posterior cusp that moves in a direction opposite to the anterior cusp at the closure point. The patient with mitral stenosis (lower panel) shows a flat diastolic configuration with no visible A wave and a posterior cusp that tends to follow the anterior in diastole. MV, mitral valve; RESP, respiration; PHONO, phonocardiogram; ECG, electrocardiogram. (From King, D. L., editor: Diagnostic ultrasound, St. Louis, 1974, The C. V. Mosby Co.)

cians able to expertly interpret the tests, are in short supply. This has been a limiting factor in both the quality of tests performed and its acceptance in a community. Because of the way echocardiography is performed, the sound wave beam samples a relatively small, select area of the cardiac structure studied or the chamber evaluated, and thus in situations where abnormalities are localized to one segment of the heart, the echocardiogram is of limited value.

Indications for echocardiography

All the disorders listed previously, or a suspicion of these disorders, would be an indication to perform an echocardiogram. The echocardiogram is indicated also in situations in which the only abnormality is a cardiac murmur heard on ausculation and the question is raised of whether this murmur is indicative of organic heart disease or just an innocent murmur.

Pitfalls

There is no contraindication to echocardiography, since there is no inherent risk in the procedure. There are, however pitfalls in the performance of the technique, such as difficulty in obtaining consistently high quality echocardiograms and in interpreting these records. Possible risk to the patient may be considered to be misdiagnosis or wrong therapeutic decisions that are based on poor quality echocardiograms. It can be unequivocally stated that poorly done echocardiography and inadequately interpreted echocardiography are worse than no echocardiography.

Phonocardiography and external pulse recording
Phonocardiography

This is the graphic recording of sounds that originate in the heart and the great vessels. This recording may be accomplished by placing microphones on the surface of the body or by introducing special apparatus into the heart (intracardiac phonocardiography). This discussion will be limited to the former.

Phonocardiography is an extension of auscultation of the heart as performed with the stethoscope, in that it generally records only the sounds that can be heard by the clinician. The phonocardiogram is, however, superior to the stethoscope in recording low frequency sounds, that is, gallop sounds, while the stethoscope is better in appreciating high frequency sounds, or murmurs. The phonocardiogram can record the four components of the first sound, systolic murmurs, the two components of the second sound (aortic and pulmonic), the opening snap of mitral stenosis, third and fourth gallop sounds, and clicks. It can also give information about *relative* loudness of these events. A normal phonocardiogram is displayed in Figs. 4-10 and 4-12.

The phonocardiogram is commonly recorded simultaneously with other external

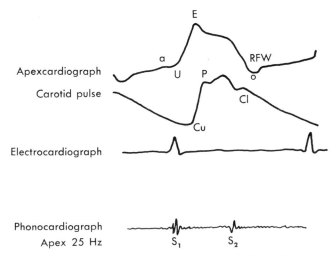

Fig. 4-12. Normal phonocardiogram and external pulse recordings displayed with the ECG.

pulses that can serve as a reference for timing various sounds. These are carotid pulse, jugular pulse, and apexcardiogram.

Carotid pulse tracing

This is the graphic recording of the displacement of the carotid artery in the neck, produced by each heartbeat and reflecting small volume changes in a segment of this artery. This recording is obtained by applying a pressure-sensitive transducer over the point of maximum pulsation of the carotid artery in the neck. Information is thus gained about the rate of rise of this curve, its duration, and its overall contour. Although records obtained in this manner closely resemble tracings obtained by pressure transducers inside the vessels, carotid pulse tracings cannot be used to measure absolute pressures. A normal carotid pulse tracing is displayed in Fig. 4-12.

Jugular pulse tracing

This is obtained in a similar manner to the carotid pulse tracing, except that the recording is obtained over the jugular venous system and yields information about events in the right atrium and right ventricle.

Apexcardiogram

This is the graphic recording of displacement of the chest wall produced by the motion of the underlying left ventricle. Analysis of this record provides information about events in this chamber. A normal apexcardiogram is displayed in Fig. 4-12.

Clinical uses

The phonocardiogram is most useful for accurate timing of various sounds and murmurs. Examples are timing the opening snap of mitral stenosis, timing the closing of aortic and pulmonic valves of the second sound (A2-P2), and evaluating clicks whether they are ejection (early in systole) or late systolic clicks. The phonocardiogram is also useful in recording the shape of various murmurs that are heard.

The carotid pulse tracing provides information about the functional state or the performance of the left ventricle. This is accomplished by measuring the various components of the curve produced on the graph. Also, general evaluation of the contour of the curve can give information about aortic stenosis, aortic insufficiency, mitral insufficiency, and idiopathic hypertrophic subaortic stenosis (IHSS).

The jugular pulse tracing, serves as a reference for the phonocardiogram, yields information about right ventricular hypertrophy, elevated pressure in the right atrium, tricuspid regurgitation, and constrictive pericarditis, and aids in the analysis of complex arrhythmias. In complete heart block it records the cannon A wave that is observed at the bedside examination.

Apex cardiography is helpful in timing various heart sounds, especially the opening snap of mitral stenosis. It is also useful as a reference tracing for locating the fourth heart sound or the atrial gallop, and in distinguishing the origin of the gallop (right or left side). The evaluation of the contour of the tracing yields information about left ventricular hypertrophy, possible aortic or mitral stenosis, or idiopathic hypertrophic subaortic stenosis.

These four tests—the phonocardiogram, carotid pulse tracing, jugular pulse tracing, and apexcardiogram—are valuable because they provide a permanent objective record far superior to handwritten descriptive records and can be used in serial comparison in the same patient. They are also superb devices for teaching the physical examination and auscultation of the heart.

Limitations

There are limitations in the clinical use of these tests. Because they serve as an extension of the physical examination, what cannot be heard through the stethoscope usually cannot be recorded on the phonocardiogram. A specific diagnosis can rarely be made *only* by inspection of these graphic methods. Another limitation is the skill and the time necessary to perform the tests. Also, information obtained is of a qualitative nature; therefore statements about quantitative events or abnormalities cannot be made.

Indications

These graphic methods are indicated whenever a permanent objective record is important as well as when the specific information about the pulses or timing of various auscultative findings is not otherwise available.

Equipment, presently available, permits the simultaneous recording and superimposition with the electrocardiogram of echocardiograms, multiple phonocardiograms, carotid pulse tracings, venous pulse tracings, and apexcardiograms. The value of the individual tests is usually enhanced when they are performed in this manner.

Nuclear cardiology

Radioactive tracer techniques are being used in cardiovascular diagnosis with increasing frequency. These tests generally qualify as "noninvasive" because they are safe and can be performed repeatedly, and the total radiation exposure is considered minimal. They do involve intravenous injection of a tracer material, but this does not involve more than the drawing of routine blood samples.

The general technique in all of these tests is the injection of a radioactive tracer material into a vein and recording the emitted radioactivity over a specific area of the body. By using various types of tracers as well as different recording techniques, vastly different types of information can be obtained. Among the diagnostic tests employing radioactive tracer techniques are lung scanning, angiocardioscan, and myocardial scanning.

Lung scanning

In lung scanning a tracer of adequate quantity is injected and subsequently trapped in the lung capillaries to obtain information about the status of pulmonary perfusion.

In scanning for right-to-left shunts, the radioactive material, instead of being trapped in the pulmonary vasculature, is passed to the left side of the heart and trapped in systemic capillaries (for example, in the kidney or the spleen), where radioactivity will be seen. In such a situation an angiocardioscan (nuclear angiocardiogram) can further localize the shunt.

The lung scan is most helpful in a diagnosis of pulmonary embolus when the x-ray film of the chest is normal or near-normal, and when the test is interpreted in conjunction with the ventilation scan, which would detect the presence of parenchymal lung disease. This is discussed on p. 100.

In the presence of grossly abnormal x-ray films of the chest resulting from parenchymal lung disease, such as those normally seen in chronic obstructive lung disease or pneumonia, the diagnostic accuracy of a lung scan is markedly diminished. In questionable or doubtful cases it is necessary to use selective pulmonary angiography to obtain a definite diagnosis. Occasionally, a lung scan will reveal absolutely no perfusion on one side of the lung. This could be the manifestation of a large pulmonary embolus or may indicate a congenitally absent or atretic right or left pulmonary artery.

Nuclear angiocardiogram (angiocardioscan)

In this test a bolus of radionuclide is injected intravenously and its course through the circulatory system is followed with a scintillation camera. The size, shape, and sequence of filling of the various chambers of the heart can then be studied. This procedure is most useful in the detection of intracardiac shunt or complex congenital heart diseases. It is also helpful in evaluating surgically performed shunt in congenital heart disease. In addition, it supplies information about cardiac size and chamber enlargement, and is helpful in diagnosis of pericardial effusion and differentiating it from cardiomegaly. Presently the echocardiogram is superior in detecting and quantitating pericardial effusion, but in difficult or doubtful cases nuclear angiocardiography is useful. It also provides information about the contour of the left ventricle, which helps in the diagnosis of left ventricular aneurysm. Recent attempts have been made in evaluating left ventricular function by calculating volumes and ejection fractions of the left ventricle. Presently the diagnostic accuracy of this method of scanning does not match that obtained by cardiac catheterization and angiocardiography with injection of dye, and therefore it remains a screening test.

Myocardial scanning

Recently radioactive tracer techniques have been used in attempts to evaluate the site and extent of myocardial infarction. This technique involves the injection of tracers, usually radioactive potassium (^{43}K), that show decreased accumulation in infarcted tissue. The usefulness of this test is extended when performed during stress of either exercise or pacing, where a relative decrease of myocardial perfusion can be detected in patients with coronary artery disease in the absence of myocardial infarction. Thus, evaluation of the size of the myocardial infarct, diagnosis of coronary artery disease, and evaluation of patency or occlusion of vein bypass grafts are making the techniques of myocardial scanning one of the most promising fields in nuclear cardiology.

Clinical value

In general, tracer techniques are inadequate or poor in the evaluation of isolated valvular lesions of mild to moderate severity or mixed valvular lesions. Although the diagnostic potential of tracer techniques is great, at the present time the main indications for tracer methods in cardiology are for the lung scan (evaluating pulmonary embolus), detecting right-to-left shunts, and screening of congenital heart disease. Because of limitations of resolution as well as limitations dictated by equipment and characteristics of various tracers, the other applications discussed either are not generally available or are still in the experimental or developmental stage.

Pacemaker evaluation

All pacemakers rely on batteries of one type or another to generate the pulse for pacing. Battery exhaustion is the most common cause of pacemaker failure. Thus the purpose of pacemaker evaluation is to obtain the longest possible use of a pacemaker pulse generator without exposing the patient to the risk of pacemaker failure. Pacemaker evaluation should, then, detect the early, unexpected pulse generator failure as well as delay the replacement in a well-functioning unit until signs of failure appear, instead of replacing all pacemakers at the arbitrary limit set by the manufacturers.

Pacemaker evaluation is performed through the use of the electrocardiogram equipped with an electrical interval counter, which measures the pulse interval and duration. The pulse interval or the pulse generator rate can also be transmitted over the telephone, and thus analysis can be performed without the patient leaving home.

There are several indicators of impending or actual battery exhaustion. Among these are changes in the pulse interval, a decrease in the amplitude of the pulse, a change in the duration of the pulse, and the failure of the sensing circuit. Analysis of these variables in conjunction with the standard electrocardiogram to detect loss of capture will permit detection of impending or actual pacemaker failure. Criteria as to when to replace the pacemaker have been proposed using the above variables, and although various centers may vary in their precise criteria, a loss of capture is considered an absolute indication for replacement.

INVASIVE DIAGNOSTIC METHODS IN CARDIOLOGY
Cardiac catheterization

Cardiac catheterization is the most definitive method of obtaining accurate diagnostic information of cardiac disorders and evaluating their severity. From the pioneer days of Forssmann in 1929, when he himself positioned a catheter in his own right atrium, to the present, this diagnostic test has been much expanded upon and the selective catheterization of all cardiac chambers, great vessels, and coronary arteries has been accomplished so frequently and successfully that it is now commonly performed in many hospitals with remarkable safety.

Method

Cardiac catheterization is performed by specially trained personnel (usually cardiologists and radiologists in cooperation) in a specially equipped cardiac catheterization laboratory where, besides equipment for diagnostic uses, complete resuscitative equipment is available.

In its simplest form the procedure includes introduction of cardiac catheters into the right side of the heart through an arm vein (basilic or cephalic vein) or a leg vein (the femoral vein). The catheter is advanced through the vena cava, the right atrium, the right ventricle, and pulmonary artery, and for a brief period further advanced and positioned in the distal pulmonary artery wedge position. On the left side of the heart the catheter is introduced through an artery, either the brachial artery in the arm or the femoral artery. It is advanced through the arterial system to the ascending aorta, through the aortic valve into the left ventricle, and if necessary to the left atrium.

Both of these routes can be approached by the cutdown technique. In this method, the veins are usually tied at the end of the procedure, while the arteries are repaired. The procedure also can be performed percutaneously, a method in which the vessels are not isolated and all catheters are introduced over guide wires and needles. From the various chambers, pressures are recorded, and blood is sampled and analyzed for its oxygen content, ordinarily during rest as well as exercise. This information coupled with measurement of the patient's oxygen consumption, which is obtained by collecting gases expired by the patient, reveals information about (1) the patient's cardiac output (the amount of blood pumped per minute), (2) the presence and size of right-to-left or left-to-right shunt within the cardiac chambers, (3) the presence and severity of stenosis (narrowing of various valves), and (4) the calculation of the resistance of the various vascular beds. Additional information is obtained using the indicator dilution test, angiography, and selective arteriography.

Indicator dilution test. An indicator is a substance that can be harmlessly introduced into the cardiovascular system and detected with appropriate sensing apparatus. The substance commonly used for determining cardiac output is indocyanine green, which is introduced on the venous side and sampled by a densitometer (an instrument that is sensitive to optical changes of the blood). Curves that are thus obtained are used to calculate cardiac output, blood flow, and shunts. A slight modification of this principle uses hydrogen gas that is introduced into the patient's system by inhalation. The gas is diffused into the circulation at the level of the pulmonary capillaries. Left-to-right shunts at various levels within the heart chambers can be detected by specially designed platinum-tipped electrode catheters positioned at specific sites.

Angiography. Angiography is a modification of the basic catheterization technique. Here the positioning of the catheter tip in a specific area of the cardiovascular system and injection of contrast substance permit opacification of the area. Concomitant x-ray filming provides a permanent graphic record. Injection of such contrast material into the right atrium is useful in detection of pericardial effusion and also for visualization of the tricuspid valve. Injection into the right or left ventricle gives information about the size and contraction of the respective chambers, as well as the tricuspid and the mitral valves. Injection into the pulmonary artery visualizes the pulmonary arterial system and is the most definitive way of diagnosing pulmonary embolus.

Selective coronary arteriography. Selective injection into the coronary arteries is called selective coronary arteriography. This technique was introduced in 1962 and has since served as the cornerstone for the evaluation of coronary artery disease and has enabled the development of surgical revascularization procedures. For selective coronary arteriography, various catheters are positioned at the coronary ostia, where dye is injected, and x-ray films are taken. Similarly, results of vein bypass grafting are evaluated by injection of dye into the graft that is interposed between the aorta and the coronary arteries.

Electrophysiologic studies can be added to standard cardiac catheterization with the use of specially-designed catheters with recording and stimulating electrodes at their tip. This technique of intracardiac electrography, sometimes referred to as His bundle recording, is useful in evaluation of atrioventricular block, supraventricular and ventricular tachyarrhythmias, and functional characteristics of the sinus and the A-V node.

Limitations

These techniques are invasive and therefore pose some discomfort as well as small but definite risks to the patient's life or well-being. In addition, the tests are costly to perform, both in manpower and equipment, and need a team of highly trained, technically capable people. Another limitation or disadvantage of the test is that the contrast medium itself can cause changes in the cardiovascular system under study.

Indications

The indications for cardiac catheterization are many and well defined. The procedure, because of its cost and inherent hazards should not be performed before careful consideration is given to the indications.

The most common indication is clinically diagnosed congenital or acquired heart disease requiring surgical therapy. In most patients noninvasive diagnostic methods are adequate in making an exact diagnosis and also in deciding on the advisability of surgery. Even in these patients, preoperative cardiac catheterization should be almost always performed to confirm the diagnosis and to evaluate cardiac function. Occasionally cardiac catheterization will reveal an unsuspected cardiac lesion and will also be helpful in determining the type of surgical procedure for the individual patient.

Cardiac catheterization is indicated for patients with heart disease of unknown etiology where an exact diagnosis would improve or change the mode of therapy.

Evaluation of operative results, another indication, applies to both congenital cardiac disease and acquired heart disease in adults. The following could thus be evaluated: the status of prosthetic valves and of shunt procedures, the results of corrective procedures for congenital heart disease, and the adequacy and patency of grafts for coronary artery disease.

Presently the largest number of catheterizations and angiograms are being performed on patients with coronary artery disease, first to diagnose the presence of coronary artery disease, and second to select patients for surgical revascularization.

Indications for selective coronary angiography are continuously being redefined but at present the commonly accepted indication is the presence of symptomatic coronary artery disease with angina pectoris that has not responded well to medical therapy. Some advocates of this catheterization technique believe that all patients with suspicion of coronary artery disease should undergo coronary angiography. An uncommon indication for cardiac catheterization is the evaluation of the cardiac status of a patient, primarily for a nonmedical reason. This includes athletes with poorly defined murmurs who need permission for unrestricted activity, or airline pilots who have vague chest pains or mild electrocardiographic abnormalities and who need complete clearance to continue flight status. Lastly, cardiac catheterization is also performed for investigative purposes on volunteers for research purposes who provide informed consent for the procedure.

Contraindications

There is no absolute contraindication for cardiac catheterization and angiography. Relative contraindications would be the presence of severe uncontrolled congestive heart failure, severe arrhythmias, and a history of allergy to the dye. An essential study under this last condition can be carried out if appropriate premedication is given and precautions are taken. Some investigators believe that contrast injections should be avoided in patients with severe pulmonary hypertension or severe aortic stenosis.

Pitfalls

Individual discussion of the pitfalls in cardiac catheterization is beyond the scope of this book. To avoid serious errors, if the diagnosis from the cardiac catheterization laboratory is at variance with the clinical diagnosis, the catheterization diagnosis should not be accepted without any question. The catheterization data, as well as the clinical data, should be critically reviewed.

Risks

Catheterization of the right side of the heart has a very small risk of essentially no mortality and a morbidity of less than 1% that is limited to arrhythmias or a minor amount of bleeding. Catheterization of the left side of the heart, combined with cardiac angiography, is somewhat more hazardous and carries the risk of myocardial infarction, cerebrovascular accident, arterial bleeding, and arterial thrombosis with possible loss of limb. The risk of death varies among hospitals. The procedure with the highest risk of death is selective coronary angiography. In this procedure the risk of mortality varies from less than 0.1% to 1% or even higher, depending on the patient population studied and the experience of the catheterization team. It is mandatory that there be a written, informed consent in the patient's record prior to the procedure.

Diagnostic pericardiocentesis

When pericardial effusion is present in large quantities or has accumulated rapidly in smaller quantities, it causes life-threatening complications of tachycardia, hypotension, and shock with elevated venous pressure (a combination characteristic of cardiac tamponade). In such a situation, a therapeutic pericardiocentesis is performed to remove fluid and relieve pressure on the heart. In some situations where pericardial fluid is present without causing cardiac tamponade, a diagnostic pericardiocentesis is performed to remove a small sample of the fluid for laboratory examination. This procedure is usually performed with the patient in a semisitting position, with a pericardiocentesis needle introduced via the subxiphoid approach into the pericardial space, under continuous electrocardiographic monitoring. The V lead of the ECG is connected to the needle and the ECG is monitored to prevent puncture of the heart. S-T segment elevation indicates needle contact with the epicardium and dictates withdrawal of the needle. The fluid removed is studied for chemical content (protein, sugar, LDH), malignant cells, infection (bacterial, fungal, tubercular, or viral), or other tests as indicated.

When echocardiography is used in the evaluation of the pericardial effusion, no air should be introduced, but if x-ray films have been used, a volume of air equal to the volume of fluid removed may be introduced to better define the pericardial space. Monitoring right atrial pressures before and after pericardiocentesis yields hemodynamic information useful in the diagnosis of cardiac tamponade or coexistent pericardial constriction.

Clinical value

Diagnostic pericardiocentesis is useful in cardiac disorders of unknown etiology when pericardial effusion is present. This diagnostic test is most helpful in situations of infection, tumor, and immunologic disorders, that is, systemic lupus erythematosus (SLE) or rheumatoid arthritis.

Limitations

Pericardiocentesis may be ineffective if pericardial effusion is loculated or mainly posterior without free-flowing anterior effusion.

Indications

The main indications for diagnostic pericardiocentesis are infective pericarditis and suspected carcinomatous infiltration of the pericardium.

Contraindications

An absolute contraindication is an uncooperative, uncontrollable patient, as this would markedly increase the risk of laceration of the heart. A bleeding disorder or anticoagulant therapy should also be considered a contraindication for elective diagnostic pericardiocentesis. Puncture of a cardiac chamber under these circumstances may precipitate uncontrollable bleeding in the pericardial sac with cardiac tamponade.

Pitfalls

Among the many pitfalls encountered in the performance of this test is the danger of puncturing and entering the right atrial chamber if the needle is directed more towards the right shoulder. In this situation elevation of the S-T segment may not be seen, but there may be elevation of the P-R interval, a clue that the right atrial chamber has been entered. Aspirated blood that clots normally and has the patient's usual hematocrit, indicates that a cardic chamber has been entered. Air should not be injected until the operator is absolutely certain that the needle is in the pericardial space and not in the cardiac chamber.

Risks

The risks of this procedure include arrhythmias (atrial or ventricular), puncture of a cardiac chamber (usually the right atrium or right ventricle), coronary arterial puncture, pneumothorax (puncture of the lung), and possible introduction of infection. With careful attention to technique and experience the risk of complications is minimal. Permission with informed consent is needed before the procedure.

Cardiac biopsy

The cardiac biopsy is probably the most invasive diagnostic test in cardiac disorders, other than open surgical exploration for diagnostic purposes. Generally two approaches are used. Transthoracic needle biopsy of the left ventricular myocardium is the older method and is generally considered to have a higher risk of complications. Percutaneous transvenous endomyocardial biopsy is a newer, safer technique in which forceps are introduced through a vein, usually the internal jugular, and through the right atrium into the right ventricle. The biopsy specimen is obtained from the right ventricular apex or the septum. A similar technique for biopsy of the left ventricular endomyocardium has also been developed.

Indications

Endomyocardial biopsy is indicated in the diagnosis of rejection of the transplanted heart, in diffuse infiltrative disorders of the heart (amyloidosis or tumors of the heart), and in small vessel disease of the endomyocardium, which is a newly discovered abnormality being studied by the biopsy method. Other conditions in which biopsy has been useful are primary myocardial disease (cardiomyopathies), hypertrophic obstructive cardiomyopathy (idiopathic hypertrophic subaortic stenosis), hypothyroidism, some of the storage diseases (glycogen storage disease), and others.

Limitations

The disease process must be diffuse to be diagnosed by the biopsy, since the sampling is very small. The transvenous endomyocardial biopsy, the more common method used, samples the right ventricle and the right ventricular septum, but does not sample the left ventricle. The risk of the procedure, although very low in initial reports, is expected to increase as the procedure is popularized and performed in more centers.

Contraindications

Bleeding disorders, anticoagulation therapy, and an uncooperative patient are among the contraindications for this procedure.

Risks

Complications of endomyocardial biopsy include right-sided pneumothorax immediately after the procedure, usually a self-limited inconsequential problem; arrhythmias, either isolated ventricular contractions, premature contractions, atrial fibrillation, flutter, or supraventricular tachycardia; in rare cases, evidence of right ventricular puncture that presents as mild pericarditis or intrapericardial bleeding. Permission is obtained as in cardiac catherization.

CHAPTER 5

Diagnostic tests for pulmonary disorders

ANATOMY AND PHYSIOLOGY

An exchange of gases between blood and air occurs within the lungs. This vital function is possible because the structure of the lungs provides open tubes (bronchi and bronchioles) that branch into millions of thin-walled air sacs (alveoli). These air sacs are in contact with the blood through the network of capillaries surrounding them. The bronchi and bronchioles are illustrated in Figs. 5-1 and 5-2. The diffusion of gases, both from the venous blood to the alveoli and from the alveoli to the capillary blood, takes place through the thin alveolar and capillary walls. Because of the tremendous number of alveoli, each well supplied with capillaries (Fig. 5-2), large amounts of oxygen diffuse very rapidly into the blood and large amounts of carbon dioxide diffuse rapidly into the alveolar spaces to be expelled during expiration.

PATHOPHYSIOLOGY (TERMINOLOGY)

Disturbances of either ventilation or perfusion can cause significant disease and incapacity in terms of pulmonary function, resulting in hypoxemia and respiratory acidosis or alkalemia. The mechanisms responsible are hyperventilation, alveolar hypoventilation, altered ventilation/perfusion ratio, venoarterial shunt (right/left shunt), and diffusion block. The last three conditions are illustrated in Fig. 5-3.

Alveolar hypoventilation

A decrease in ventilation to a large number of alveoli is present in this condition. This decrease is defined by a rise in arterial carbon dioxide (PCO_2). Attendent to it will be decreased arterial PO_2 and acidosis.

Abnormal ventilation/perfusion ratio (V/Q)

Marked decrease in ventilation/perfusion ratio (Fig. 5-4) results from marked hypoventilation in relation to perfusion. The opposite, marked decrease in perfusion to ventilation, causes an increased ventilation/perfusion ratio. This is mainly reflected by an increase in residual volume. Both of the above abnormalities occur in chronic obstructive lung disease.

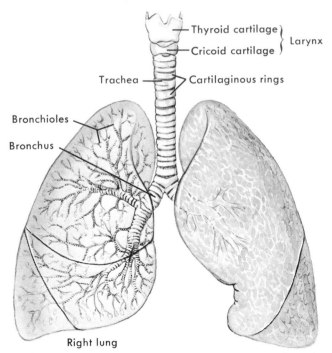

Fig. 5-1. The respiratory tract with the right lung cut away to expose bronchi and bronchioles. (From Schottelius, B. A., and Schottelius, D. D.: Textbook of physiology, ed. 17, St. Louis, 1973, The C. V. Mosby Co.)

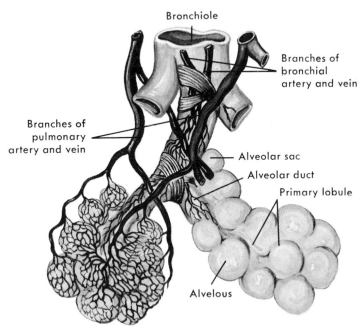

Fig. 5-2. The capillary network surrounding the alveoli. (From Schottelius, B. A., and Schottelius, D. D.: Textbook of physiology, ed. 17, St. Louis, 1973, The C. V. Mosby Co.)

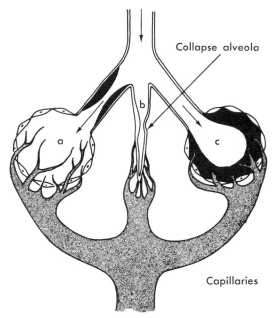

Fig. 5-3. **a**, Altered ventilation/perfusion ratio; **b**, arteriovenous shunt (right/left shunt); **c**, diffusion block.

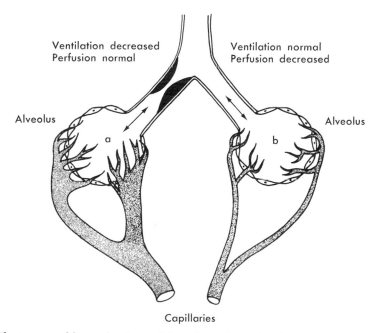

Fig. 5-4. The two possible mechanisms of altered ventilation/perfusion ratio. **a**, Increased perfusion to poorly ventilated alveoli; **b**, decreased perfusion to normally ventilated alveoli.

Arteriovenous shunt (right-to-left shunt)

This term means that the blood from the right side of the heart will be shunted to the left side without having been oxygenated and without having given up its carbon dioxide. The mechanism of this condition is illustrated in Fig. 5-5. It will be noted when comparing Fig. 5-5 with Fig. 5-4 that the difference between ventilation/perfusion abnormalities and right-to-left shunt is determined by the size of the shunt. The mechanisms responsible are the same.

Diffusion block

This term implies a physiochemical interference with the rate of gas exchange across the alveolar-capillary membrane. Since carbon dioxide diffuses almost twenty times faster than O_2, hypoxemia is usually the result, with arterial P_{CO_2} unaffected.

LABORATORY TESTS

In addition to the pulmonary function disorders, there are usually associated structural changes. Hence, diagnostic tests for evaluating pulmonary function are varied for detection of anatomical anomalies, infectious processes, physiological disturbances, or a combination of all three.

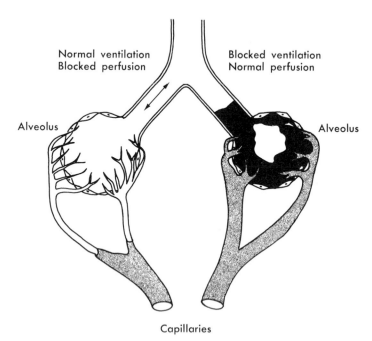

Fig. 5-5. Arteriovenous shunt (right to left shunt).

Chest roentgenography

Chest roentgenography is a valuable addition to the physical examination because it initiates the diagnostic search by revealing an abnormality in an asymptomatic individual, detecting pulmonary involvement in ill patients, and providing a guide to the selection of subsequent diagnostic procedures. Fluoroscopy and tomography are special radiographic techniques that may provide diagnostic insights.

Fluoroscopy permits visualization of inspiration and expiration. It helps in localizing lesions and in determining whether they are pulsatile or not. It also gives information about diaphragmatic movement.

Tomography (laminography) consists of a sequence of x-ray films, each representing a slice of the lung at different depths. This procedure is useful in identifying the presence of calcium or a cavity within a lesion, the presence of hilar adenopathy, tracheal or broncheal abnormalities, and the shape of mediastinal masses.

Sputum examination

The sputum examination is also quite commonly employed, in identifying specific infectious agents so that proper therapy may be instituted. Stained smears of the sputum may help in identification of the causative organism in many bacterial pneumonias, tuberculosis, and some fungous infections. That the specimen be really sputum and not saliva is important. Transtracheal aspiration of sputum will eliminate the oral contamination of normal flora.

Table 5-1. Normal pulmonary function tests

	Age		
Test	*20-39*	*40-59*	*60+*
VC (liters)			
Men	3.35-5.90	2.72-5.30	2.42-4.70
Women	2.45-4.38	2.09-4.02	1.91-3.66
FEV$_1$L			
Men	3.11-4.64	2.45-3.98	2.09-3.32
Women	2.16-3.65	1.60-3.09	1.30-2.53
FEV% (FEV/VC)			
Men	77	70	60
Women	82	77	74
Residual volume (liters)			
Men	1.13-2.32	1.45-2.62	1.77-2.77
Women	1.00-2.00	1.16-2.20	1.32-2.40
Total lung capacity (liters)			
Men	4.80-7.92	4.50-7.62	4.35-7.32
Women	3.61-6.18	3.41-6.02	3.31-5.86

Pulmonary function tests

Pulmonary function tests measure the flow of air in and out of the lungs, diffusing capacity, lung compliance, and so forth. They also provide valuable information about functional aberrations resulting from obstruction or diffusion changes. Normal values for pulmonary function tests are displayed in Table 5-1.

Vital capacity (VC) is the total volume of air exhaled after a full inspiration and forced expiration. Normally 80% of this volume is exhaled in one second and is called the *forced expiratory volume (FEV$_1$)*. In obstructive lung disease the patient is unable to breathe out fully and therefore the vital capacity and the FEV$_1$ are both reduced, as is the FEV/VC%. In restrictive lung disease the chest cannot expand fully and therefore the vital capacity is low. There is decrease in lung compliance. However, airway resistance is normal and the FEV$_1$ is therefore not reduced proportionately, causing the FEV/VC% to be normal or high (Fig. 5-6).

Residual volume represents the air that cannot be removed from the lungs, even by forceful expiration. One technique for measuring the residual volume is through the use of a body plethysmograph and another is a helium dilution test in which the patient is connected to a spirometer circuit containing helium. After several minutes of rebreathing, the degree of dilution of helium is measured.

Total lung capacity represents the volume to which the lungs can be expanded with greatest inspiratory effort.

Blood gases

Blood gases are analyzed to determine the oxygen and acid-base status of the patient and are usually measured on arterial blood.

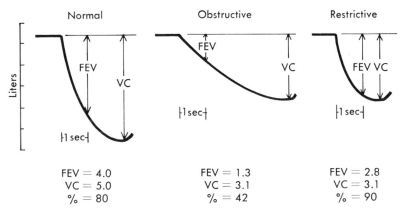

Fig. 5-6. Measurement of the forced expiratory volume, FEV$_1$, and vital capacity, VC. The patient makes a full inspiration and then exhales as hard and as fast as possible. As the patient exhales, the pen moves down. The FEV$_1$ is the volume exhaled in one sec; the VC is the total volume exhaled. Note the differences among the normal, obstructive, and restrictive patterns. (From West, J. B.: Disturbances of respiratory function. In Harrison's Principles of internal medicine, ed. 7, New York, 1974, McGraw-Hill Book Co.)

NORMAL BLOOD GAS VALUES

	Arterial blood	*Mixed venous blood*
pH	7.40 (7.35-7.45)	7.36 (7.3-7.41)
Po_2	80-100 mm Hg	35-40 mm Hg
O_2 Sat	95%	70%-75%
Pco_2	35-45 mm Hg	41-51 mm Hg
HCO_3	22-26 mEq/l	22-26 mEq/l
Base excess (BE)	−2 to +2	−2 to +2

The pH measures the acidity or alkalinity of the blood. A low pH indicates acidemia. A high pH indicates alkalemia.

The Po_2 measures the pressure exerted by the small amount of oxygen dissolved in the plasma. Most of the oxygen in the blood is carried by the hemoglobin.

O_2 saturation (Sat) of hemoglobin is a measure of the percentage of oxygen that the hemoglobin is carrying related to the total amount the hemoglobin could carry.

The Pco_2, influenced by the lungs, measures the pressure exerted by dissolved CO_2 in the blood. An elevated Pco_2 indicates respiratory acidosis due to hypoventilation or metabolic alkalosis due to a loss of H^+ and Cl from body fluids, the gastrointestinal tract, and the kidneys, and retention of HCO_3 through the kidneys. A depressed Pco_2 indicates respiratory alkalosis resulting from hyperventilation or secondary hyperventilation resulting from metabolic acidosis.

HCO_3 (bicarbonate) and base excess are influenced by metabolic changes. Bicarbonate is an alkaline substance, and the term "excess base" refers to bicarbonate as well as other bases in the blood. An elevation in this parameter indicates metabolic alkalosis; a depression indicates metabolic acidosis.

Sometimes in order to evaluate the exact metabolic state of the patient, one must determine arterial blood gases, pH, and serum electrolytes. For example, a mild case of hypokalemic alkalosis along with respiratory acidosis may give normal arterial blood gases and pH. Unless one is aware of this interrelationship and measures the electrolytes along with the blood gases, one may never be able to detect the mild hypokalemic alkalosis and thus the presence of respiratory acidosis, the balance of which gives the false normal acid-base status.

Pleural fluid examination

Pleural fluid is easily accessible for examination by means of a diagnostic thoracentesis. When present, it may be secondary to and confirm the diagnosis of cancer, tuberculosis, or other infections and pancreatitis or rheumatoid arthritis.

Normally the pleural cavity is a potential space with moist membranes but no fluid present. However, in certain disease conditions fluid may accumulate in the pleural cavity creating a real space.

Pleural fluid consists of either transudates or exudates. *Transudates* pass through a membrane or are extruded from tissue, such as would occur in congestive heart failure, cirrhosis of the liver, and nephritis. *Exudates* are composed of thicker cellular fluid that has escaped from blood vessels, such as would occur with inflammation and infection of the pleura. Accordingly, the protein content of exudates is high compared with transudates.

Whenever there is doubt as to whether pleural fluid is exudate or transudate, it is essential that a small amount be aspirated and that the protein content be measured. The procedure is nontraumatic to the patient and easy to perform. If the protein content is above 2.5 gm%, it is exudative effusion; if less than 2.5 gm%, it is transudative.

The most common cause of transudates is congestive heart failure. The most common causes of exudates, which are nonbloody, are infections and inflammations. *Tuberculous pleuritis* should always be considered in exudative, nonbloody pleural effusion. The easiest and quickest way of making a diagnosis in this case is by a closed needle pleural biopsy, which shows the caseating granuloma. Bacteriologic culture of the pleural fluid is also important. However, it takes two to three weeks for the growth of the tubercle organism.

Acute pancreatitis can cause pleural effusion. In this case the elevated amylase level in the pleural fluid will be diagnostic of the condition. Other subdiaphragmatic inflammatory processes can also cause effusions, which in the early stages are usually sterile transudates.

Another example of pleural effusion is *Meig's syndrome*, which is usually transudate and is associated with carcinoma of the ovaries.

Diagnostic clues from appearance of pleural fluid

If the effusion has a milky appearance the presence of chyle is indicated and obstruction or rupture of the thoracic duct is implicated.

Hemorrhagic pleural fluid indicates either carcinoma or pulmonary embolus.

Overtly purulent fluid in the pleural cavity is called empyema. A gram stain and culture should be performed in such a case so that the patient may be managed properly. In rare occasions the tuberculous effusion may resemble empyema, which is sometimes the result of the secondary bacterial infection of the tuberculous process.

Pulmonary perfusion scan

Pulmonary perfusion scans are of minimal risk and discomfort to the patient. Perfusion scans have been particularly helpful in detecting zones of decreased or absent blood flow compatible with pulmonary embolism.

Ventilation scan

A ventilation scan is made following the inhalation of a radioactive gas. If a perfusion defect is the result of embolism, ventilation will be intact and alveolar dead space visualized. If the perfusion abnormality is the result of obstructive lung disease, defective ventilation will also be present.

Bronchoscopy

Bronchoscopy permits visualization of the trachea and its major subdivisions. Biopsy material may also be obtained through the bronchoscopy tube.

Bronchography

Bronchography involves the use of radiopaque material that is instilled into the tracheobronchial tree through a catheter. All of the tracheobronchial tree can then be seen on x-ray films. Diagnoses possible with the use of bronchography include bronchiectasis, obstruction in distal bronchi, and tracheobronchial malformation.

Pulmonary angiography

Pulmonary angiography permits visualization of the pulmonary circulation. The dye is introduced into the circulation through a systemic vein, the right ventricle, or the pulmonary artery, and a film records the distribution of the dye. This procedure is useful in detecting pulmonary emboli and lesions of the pulmonary vasculature, particularly if it is done by selective pulmonary angiography, that is, separate injection of the right and left pulmonary arteries.

Mediastinoscopy

Mediastinoscopy visualizes the mediastinal space, and a biopsy may be taken. A lighted scope is inserted through an incision at the suprasternal notch.

Lung biopsy

Ultimately, in certain situations, a lung biopsy may be necessary to the diagnosis, and can be performed by either closed needle or small thoracotomy procedures. The specimen obtained is both cultured and processed for pathologic examination.

Kveim skin test and biopsy

The Kveim test is a reliable means of confirming the diagnosis of sarcoidosis. The test consists of an intradermal inoculation of an antigen composed of human sarcoidal tissue. The development of a papule in four to six weeks is considered a positive reaction. On biopsy the papule shows the typical noncaseating granulomas of sarcoidosis. This test has been shown to give positive results in the majority of cases, with less than 3% false positives. The Kveim test is particularly valuable when biopsy cannot be performed because of the absence of enlarged lymph nodes or if, when a biopsy is taken, the granulomas obtained are nonspecific.

LABORATORY TESTS IN THE CLINICAL SETTING
Chronic obstructive pulmonary disease

Chronic obstructive pulmonary disease is one of the most disabling diseases and involves a diminution of the flow rate of air from the lungs resulting from airway narrowing. It is divided into three major categories: emphysema, bronchitis, and asthma.

Laboratory tests

The most commonly employed test for assessing the diseases in this category is the FEV_1. FEV_1 levels are reduced, as are the VC and FEV/VC% Residual volume is increased as a correlative to diminished vital capacity. Additionally, the arterial blood gases reveal hypoxemia, with the PO_2 less than 70 mm Hg.

Differential diagnosis

Functionally the differences between pure emphysema and pure bronchitis are as follows. In pure emphysema, total lung capacity and the residual volume are increased much more than they are in pure bronchitis, in which the total lung capacity is often normal.

In the early stages of pure emphysema the arterial PCO_2 is normal due to an increase in ventilation that compensates for the decreased PO_2. There is a marked diminution of the ratio of forced expiratory volume to vital capacity (FEV/VC). Usually this is associated with a decrease in antitrypsin titers in the blood. In contrast, pure bronchitis usually is characterized by chronic productive cough and wheezing. However, this is usually associated with hypercapnia and hypoventilation. Most commonly the hypoventilation is a result of significant ventilation perfusion inequality.

Sometimes the obstructive features of chronic lung disease may be of pure asthmatic origin; that is, spasm of the respiratory tree. In such a situation the condition will be demonstrated and will be 100% reversible with bronchodilators. This reversibility is the main characteristic of asthma, which is usually more of an acute process.

Restrictive lung disease

Restrictive lung disease includes all of the lung diseases in which the main pathophysiology is a disturbance of the diffusion of gases (diffusion block).

Laboratory tests

In restrictive lung disease, the FEV_1 is normal but the VC is reduced. However, because of the normal or even increased FEV_1, the FEV/VC% is high. This is one of the most distinguishing features differentiating restrictive lung disease from obstructive lung disease (Fig. 5-6). Also, because of the diffusion problem, partial O_2 pressure is lowered. However, because the patient naturally compensates with hyperventilation in an effort to improve the oxygen status, the pulmonary CO_2 pressure is also low. An altered ventilation perfusion ratio of varying degrees may be present, depending on the etiology.

Differential diagnosis

The diseases in the restrictive lung disease category are mostly diffuse and infiltrative. Because the clinical manifestations and physiologic abnormalities of all of them are very similar, the only way of making a differential diagnosis is by lung biopsy. This may also be necessary in some cases for more specific management. The causes of restrictive lung diseases are as follows:

1. Infections such as bacteria, fungi, and parasites, and the viruses of influenza, chickenpox, and measles
2. Neoplastic
3. Metabolic (uremic pneumonitis)
4. Physical agents such as blast or heat injury, oxygen toxicity, or postirradiation fibrosis
5. Hereditary infiltrative diseases such as cystic fibrosis, familial idiopathic pulmonary fibrosis, and neurofibromatosis
6. Circulatory disorders such as multiple pulmonary emboli, fat embolism, lymphangiography, sickle cell anemia, foreign body vasculitis from parasites or drug addiction, pulmonary edema, and chronic passive congestion with fibrosis
7. Immunologic disorders such as occur with hypersensitivity pneumonias, collagen diseases, and Goodpasture's syndrome
8. Occupational causes such as mineral dusts and chemical fumes
9. Sarcoidosis
10. Histiocytosis X
11. Idiopathic pulmonary hemosiderosis
12. Pulmonary alveolar proteinosis
13. Desquamative interstitial pneumonia

Bronchiectasis

Bronchiectasis involves weakening of the bronchial wall structures, with subsequent dilation and secondary infections.

Laboratory tests

Bronchography is the usual diagnostic tool since the diagnosis of bronchiectasis depends on demonstrating the abnormal anatomy of the bronchial system.

The most common causative organisms are *Diplococcus pneumoniae, Hemophilus influenzae,* and *Bacteroides.* If the patient has had prior antibacterial therapy, superimposed staphylococcus or pseudomonas organisms may be involved.

Lung abscess
Laboratory tests

Lung abscess is diagnosed by x-ray films of the chest that may show a solid shadow or, if certain gas-forming organisms are present, may show an air-fluid level in the lung where the abscess is located.

Identification of the organism is essential and is accomplished by culture and microscopic examination of the sputum. If the sputum specimen cannot be obtained through the usual means, bronchoscopy should be performed to obtain it. Occasionally bacteremia might occur, in which case blood cultures are of help.

Hypoventilation
Laboratory tests

Evidence of elevated arterial carbon dioxide pressure (PCO_2) should suggest the diagnosis of hypoventilation.

Differential diagnosis

The most common cause of hypoventilation is chronic obstructive lung disease. Other causes include:

1. *Deformities of the chest wall,* which are apparent to the astute observer and which include significant kyphoscoliosis and Marie-Strümpell disease (ankylosing spondylitis).
2. *Myogenic diseases* of the respiratory system such as myasthenia gravis and other myopathies.
3. *Metabolic alkalosis* in which there is marked muscle weakness. Since the PCO_2 is elevated regardless of the cause of hypoventilation, the differential diagnosis of a disproportional elevation of PCO_2 in relation to the arterial pH confirms metabolic alkalosis as a cause.
4. *"The pickwickian syndrome,"* which is extreme obesity associated with hypo-ventilation.

Hyperventilation

Hyperventilation is characterized by rapid and deep respirations. If these respirations result from anxiety, respiratory alkalosis is produced and called the hyperventilation syndrome. Hyperventilation my be secondary to metabolic acidosis and, as such, is a compensatory mechanism.

Acid-base imbalance

The following is a summary of blood gases as seen in the various states of acid-base imbalance.

	Respiratory			Metabolic		
	pH	PCO_2	HCO_3	pH	PCO_2	HCO_3
Acidosis	↓	↑	↑	↓	↓	↓
Alkalosis	↑	↓	↓	↑	↑	↑

Metabolic alkalosis is usually associated with low serum potassium and low serum chloride.

Metabolic acidosis is usually associated with hyperkalemia. Most frequently the chloride is within normal range except in renal tubular acidosis. An elevated serum chloride, then, differentiates renal tubular acidosis from other types of metabolic acidosis.

Sometimes respiratory and metabolic imbalances cancel each other and reflect normal electrolyte levels and normal blood gases. However, this does not necessarily mean that the patient's overall acid-base balance is normal. For example, a patient with a hypokalemic-chloremic metabolic alkalosis associated with respiratory acidosis may have a perfectly normal blood pH and serum potassium. But the HCO_3 and PCO_2 both are extremely elevated in both respiratory acidosis and metabolic alkalosis. Therefore, if this elevation is accompanied by normal serum potassium and blood pH, the patient's metabolic state is probably not normal.

Pulmonary embolism

Complete or partial obstruction of the pulmonary arterial blood flow results in ventilation without perfusion, or "dead space" in the lungs; atelectasis due to the loss of alveolar surfactant, a lipoprotein that maintains alveolar integrity; and a loss of vascular capacity, which, if marked, may lead to pulmonary hypertension and right heart failure.

The definitive diagnosis of pulmonary embolism requires angiographic demonstration of occlusion of the major pulmonary arteries or arterioles. However, since angiography is an invasive method, the next best diagnostic test is the *perfusion scan*. Since this test may give false positive results in the presence of chronic obstructive lung disease, it is usually combined with the *ventilation scan*, a combination that permits recognition of conditions that could not be diagnosed with only one of the tests (see p. 100).

Occasionally the *electrocardiogram* is of help in the diagnosis of pulmonary embolism. With extensive embolization there may be right axis deviation and evidence of right ventricular hypertrophy or strain, which will manifest itself with inverted T waves in the anterior precordial leads and with various arrhythmias. However, these changes are far too nonspecific for serious consideration.

The triad of bilirubinemia, elevated serum lactic dehydrogenase (LDH), and normal serum glutamic oxalacetic transaminase (SGOT) is seldom encountered and of limited value.

Carcinoma of the lung
Laboratory tests

X-ray examination of the chest is the most important initial diagnostic tool in carcinoma of the lung. Many times the patient is completely asymptomatic and the routine x-ray film reveals the nodule. After the identification of the node, serial laminograms are obtained to visualize possible calcification, which helps in the diagnosis of granuloma versus carcinoma but does not necessarily rule out either.

Bronchoscopy with bronchoscopic biopsy and, if possible, bronchoscopic aspiration for cytology, is of help, particularly in medially located pulmonary carcinoma.

Scalene node biopsy is helpful when the lung cancer is inaccessible by bronchoscopy. The scalene fat pad contains lymph nodes that receive lymphatic drainage from the lungs. Therefore, a biopsy from this area often discloses carcinoma of the lungs, granulomatous infections, and sarcoidosis.

Sputum cytology can be helpful but the results depend on the laboratory.

The positive yield in cases of lung carcinoma ranges between 30% and 70%, depending on the eagerness and expertise of the pathologist.

Needle biopsy is useful when the lesion is peripheral and nonresectable and provides a tissue diagnosis before the institution of radiation and/or chemotherapy.

Thoracentesis and *needle biopsy of the pleura* should be performed in the presence of pleural fluid. The pleural fluid exudate is usually bloody. Fluid cytology may yield the diagnosis.

Mediastinoscopy is a very good method for visualizing the lymph nodes and obtaining a biopsy of the accessible ones.

Hypersensitivity eosinophilic pneumonias

In these conditions the alveoli are filled with large mononuclear cells and eosinophils. The lung tissue is infiltrated with large numbers of eosinophils, mononuclear cells, and plasma cells.

Laboratory tests

Chest roentgenography shows patchy penumonia associated with sputum eosinophilia and/or blood eosinophilia. When the condition is acute and temporary these procedures are diagnostic. However sometimes, when the condition is recurrent and progresses to chronicity, it results in restrictive lung disease and may require *lung biopsy* for a definitive diagnosis.

CHAPTER 6

Diagnostic tests for renal disorders

ANATOMY AND PHYSIOLOGY

The functioning unit of the kidney is the nephron. There are approximately a million nephrons in each kidney. Each nephron is composed of two major units: the tubule and the gomerulus. The tubule has a blind end that begins in the cortex of the kidney (Fig. 6-1). From there its path is tortuous, bending back on itself, in a section called the *first* or *proximal convoluted tubule*. The tubule then plunges down into the medulla, where its course is smooth, and then bends back to return to the cortex. The loop thus formed is called the *loop of Henle*. Within the cortex again, the tubule twists and turns in a section known as the *second* or *distal convoluted tubule* (Fig. 6-2). It finally joins the *collecting tubule*, which ends in the pelvis of the kidney.

The glomerulus is a tuft of up to fifty capillaries that begin with an afferent arteriole and end with an efferent arteriole (Fig. 6-2). The glomerulus is invaginated into the blind upper end of the tubule. The little sac thus formed is *Bowman's capsule*. The pressure of the blood within the glomerular capillaries causes the blood to be filtered into Bowman's capsule, where it begins to pass down the tubule. As the blood filtrate passes through the tubules, it is further modified by the processes of reabsorption and secretion. All substances useful to the body are reabsorbed while hydrogen ions and ammonia are secreted.

Because of their size, red blood cells and protein do not normally pass through the glomerular filter. Thus the fluid in Bowman's capsule is a protein-free filtrate of blood plasma. Capillary permeability is increased in many renal diseases, permitting plasma proteins to pass into the urine. Also, the glomerular membrane may be so injured by disease that it fails to function as a filter, permitting blood cells and plasma protein to leak through the injured capillary to be excreted in the urine.

The glomerulus is not the only capillary bed supplying the nephron. The efferent arteriole leaving Bowman's capsule goes on to form another capillary bed, this time a low pressure bed that supplies the tubules. This low pressure in the peritubular

107

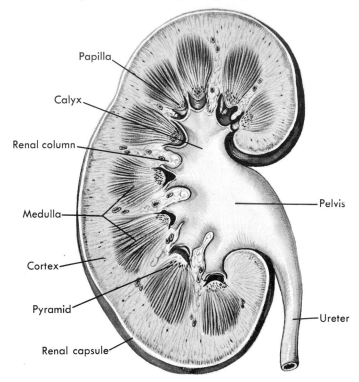

Fig. 6-1. Coronal section through the right kidney. (From Anthony, C. P., and Kolthoff, N. J.: Textbook of anatomy and physiology, ed. 9, St. Louis, 1975, The C. V. Mosby Co.)

capillary system causes it to function in much the same way as the venous ends of the tissue capillaries, with fluid being absorbed continually into the capillaries.

The effect of hormones on tubular reabsorption
Aldosterone

The adrenal corticosteroids, particularly aldosterone, have the effect of favoring the reabsorption of sodium and the excretion of potassium. The kidneys require aldosterone for the normal reabsorption of sodium. An increase in serum sodium triggers a decrease in the rate of aldosterone secretion, causing the kidney to excrete large quantities of sodium until the serum sodium is back to normal. As the serum sodium level returns to normal the rate of aldosterone secretion rises to normal. Conversely, if the serum sodium level falls considerably below normal or if the potassium rises, the rate of aldosterone secretion rises.

In adrenocortical insufficiences, such as Addison's disease, there is an excess loss of sodium whereas potassium is retained. Hyperactivity of the adrenal cortex or administration of adrenocortical hormones produces excess reabsorption of sodium and urinary loss of potassium.

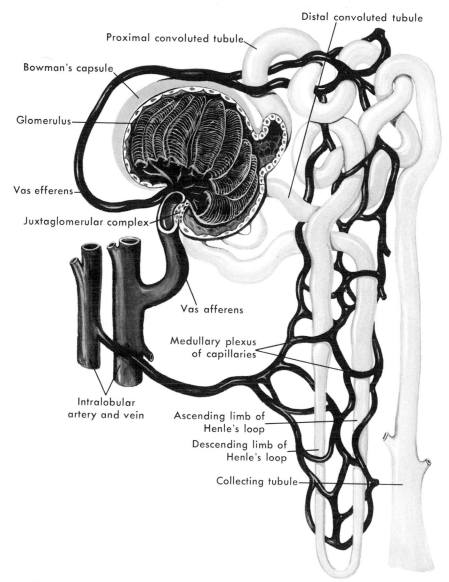

Fig. 6-2. The nephron and its blood supply. The wall of Bowman's capsule has been cut away to reveal the detail of the glomerulus. (From Schottelius, B. A., and Schottelius, D. D.: Textbook of physiology, ed. 17, St. Louis, 1973, The C. V. Mosby Co.)

Antidiuretic hormone (ADH)

The antidiuretic hormone is secreted by the hypothalamus and posterior pituitary gland. It promotes increased water reabsorption from the distal tubules and collecting ducts. ADH-controlled water reabsorption is in accord with the body's need for water, occurring independently of active solute transports. It is, therefore, called facultative reabsorption.

The renal pressor system
Renin-angiotensin

When there is a decrease in blood flow to the kidney or when extracellular sodium is low, the kidney secretes an enzyme called renin, which acts as a catalyst on one of the plasma proteins to produce a substance called angiotensin I and angiotensin II. Angiotensin has two effects: it is the most potent vasoconstrictor known and it causes increased production of aldosterone by the adrenal cortex. Aldosterone causes sodium and water retention by acting on the kidney tubules. Thus, arterial pressure is elevated by increasing the blood volume and by vasoconstriction.

PATHOPHYSIOLOGY

The functioning nephron is made of glomerular, tubular, and interstitial tissue. Therefore, although a disease state may begin in a local spot, if it progresses it ultimately involves the whole kidney because the processes in the tubular system are dependent upon the production of a filtrate by the glomerulus. If the glomerulus is involved initially in a disease and becomes grossly abnormal with decreased perfusion and filtration, ultimately the tubules show varying degrees of atrophy or fibrosis. This results in end-stage glomerular nephritis when the patient initially had an acute poststreptococcal proliferative lesion involving solely the glomerulus.

LABORATORY TESTS FOR RENAL FUNCTION

The following tests are employed in evaluating the two main functions of the kidney, glomerular filtration and tubular reabsorption.

Glomerular filtration tests

Glomerular filtration is evaluated through clearance tests that measure the rate at which certain substances are cleared from the plasma. The testing substance must be freely filtered and neither reabsorbed nor secreted by the tubules for a true picture of glomerular filtration rate, which is usually 105 to 135 ml/min.

Inulin clearance test

Inulin is a polysaccharide that is neither reabsorbed nor secreted. It is completely cleared by the kidney and is, therefore, the best indicator of glomerular function. However, because exact timing of specimen collection is required, it is not used as often as is the easy-to-perform creatinine clearance test.

NORMAL INULIN CLEARANCE (corrected to 1.73 sq m of body surface)

Males: 124 ± 25.8 ml/min
Females: 119 ± 12.8 ml/min

Creatinine clearance test

Creatinine is an endogenous waste product that is produced relative to muscle mass, and is therefore constant in an individual. Creatinine clearance is equal to glomerular filtration rate since it is excreted by glomerular filtration and is not reabsorbed or secreted by the tubule cells. The serum creatinine level, then, rises when the glomerular filtration rate falls. At the same time the creatinine clearance rate, determined on a twenty four-hour urine specimen, is low. The blood urea nitrogen (BUN) is also a rough guide to glomerular function.

NORMAL CREATININE CLEARANCE

115 ± 20 ml/min

Urea clearance test

Although urea is freely filtered by the glomeruli, it then diffuses across the nephron epithelium, causing its clearance to be considerably less than the glomerular filtration rate. Creatinine clearance tests are more practical to perform than urea clearance tests, and provide information that is easier to interpret.

Tubular function tests

Clinically, tubular function is best measured by tests that determine the ability of the tubules to concentrate and dilute the urine. Tests of urinary dilution are not as sensitive in the detection of renal disease as are tests of urinary concentration. This is especially valuable since the first function to be lost in renal disease is the ability of the kidney to concentrate urine.

Since the concentration of urine occurs in the renal medulla (interstitial fluids, loops of Henle, capillaries of the medulla, and collecting tubules), the disease processes that disturb the function or structure of the medulla produce early impairment of the concentrating ability of the kidney. Such diseases are acute tubular necrosis, obstructive uropathy, pyelonephritis, papillary necrosis, medullary cysts, hypokalemic and hypercalcemic nephropathy, and sickle cell disease.

In azotemic patients, because of disturbed glomerular and tubular function, subjection to prolonged dehydration and/or being challenged with an excess amount of water may be hazardous.

Specific gravity

This is a relatively simple and inexpensive concentration and dilution test that was discussed in Chapter 2 as a routine screening test.

Urine and serum osmolality

The measurement of urine osmolality is a more refined and accurate test for the diluting and concentrating ability of the kidneys. Osmolality is an expression of the total number of particles in a solution. Plasma osmolality is the main regulator of the release of antidiuretic hormone (ADH). When sufficient water is not being taken in, the osmolality of the plasma rises, ADH is released from the pituitary gland, and the kidneys respond by reabsorbing water from the distal tubules and producing a more concentrated urine. The converse occurs with excessive water ingestion. With the decrease in plasma osmolality, ADH is not released and the urine becomes more dilute. The normal urine osmolality depends upon the clinical setting since normally, with maximum ADH stimulation, it can be as much as 1200 mOsm/kg of body weight and with maximum ADH suppression as little as 50 mOsm/kg.

Simultaneous determination of serum and urine osmolality is often valuable in assessing the distal tubular response to circulating ADH. For example, if the patient's serum is hyperosmolar or in the upper limits of normal ranges, and the patient's urine osmolality measured at the same time is much lower, a decreased responsiveness of the distal tubules to circulating ADH is indicated.

NORMAL URINE OSMOLALITY

50-1400 mOsm/l (range)
500-800 mOsm/l (random specimen)

NORMAL SERUM OSMOLALITY

280-295 mOsm/l (range)

Phenolsulfonphthalein (PSP) excretion test

Intravenous PSP is secreted by the proximal tubules at a rate proportional to renal blood flow. If renal blood flow and proximal tubular function are normal, 28% to 35% of the PSP will be excreted in the first fifteen minutes after the IV injection.

The pitfalls of the test include incomplete emptying of the bladder and inadequate urine volumes. These can be avoided by giving the patient an excessive amount of water before the test and then injecting the dye only after the patient feels the urge to void.

Since even kidneys with markedly diminished renal blood flow will excrete a relatively normal amount of PSP in one or two hours, the first fifteen minutes of the test is the most sensitive measure of renal blood flow.

General evaluative tests for kidney function

Intravenous pyelogram (IVP)

The intravenous pyelogram is a radiologic procedure that involves the use of an intravenous injection of a contrast medium, most of which is secreted by the tubules and then concentrated. Films are then made five, ten, and fifteen minutes after injection.

This test delineates the urinary tract and thus provides information about the integrity of the kidneys, the ureters, and the bladder. It also sometimes indirectly gives information about retroperitoneal masses, which will shift the ureters.

If the patient has mild azotemia with a BUN of 40 to 50, a routine IVP may not be successful. In these situations, an infusion IVP may be considered.

Timed sequence IVP. This test is a modification of the standard IVP in which films are made every minute for five minutes after injection of the contrast medium. The difference between the times of excretion of the dye from the two kidneys indicates unilateral kidney disease. In such a case, the normal kidney shows some concentration of the dye before the abnormal one does.

It should be noted, however, that although this test is the best screening test for hypertension secondary to unilateral kidney disease, it does not differentiate between renal artery stenosis and chronic pyelonephritis or nephrosclerosis. If the patient has hypertension, the test does not differentiate between hypertension resulting from renal parenchymal disease or diffuse small vessel disease and hypertension caused by a major renal vascular obstruction.

Retrograde pyelography

Retrograde pyelography provides further information about the pelvic-calyceal system and bladder. A catheter is inserted through the urethra into each kidney pelvis. A dye is then injected that visualizes the pelvic calyces and ureteral and bladder outlines on x-ray films.

Renal angiography

Renal angiography confirms the diagnosis of renal artery stenosis after screening tests have demonstrated renal abnormality.

After percutaneous catheterization of one of the femoral arteries, the catheter is advanced to the level of the renal arteries and a radiopaque dye is injected. The passage of the dye is then monitored by x-ray techniques. If a vascular lesion is present, this procedure will demonstrate it and indicate its anatomical position.

Renal biopsy

Percutaneous biopsy of the kidney yields histologic and microscopic information about both the glomeruli and the tubules, and thus may distinguish among the causes of the nephrotic syndrome. This test is essential in the management of patients with the nephrotic syndrome in whom treatment with steroids is contemplated, since it permits a distinction between those types of nephrotic syndrome that may or may not respond to steroids. This procedure should be avoided if the patient has bleeding tendencies, uremia, or severe hypertension.

Urine culture

Urine culture and sensitivity should be ordered in genitourinary infection. In this test the colony count is important. Fewer than 10,000 viable bacterial units per milliliter are probably of no significance. If 10,000 to 100,000 colonies are cultured, no positive conclusion can be drawn. There should be over 100,000 colonies before the infection is considered significant. However, samples of urine from the ureters and renal pelvis might contain fewer bacteria and still indicate infection, because bacteria multiply while the urine is being held in the bladder.

In the absence of symptoms, a positive urine culture should elicit an inquiry into how the specimen was collected. Unless it is a catheterized or midstream voided specimen with proper cleansing of the genitalia, contamination will occur.

It should also be remembered that a negative urine culture does not necessarily rule out chronic low-grade pyelonephritis.

The Howard test

The Howard test is used to pinpoint the affected kidney in hypertension resulting from unilateral kidney disease. Ureteral catheters are placed to collect urine independently from each kidney. The seperate specimens are then analyzed for electrolytes and volume. Unilateral reduction of sodium content over 15% and/or unilateral reduction of volume over 50% is suggestive of unilateral renal disease.

The main pitfall of the test is the technical difficulty of bilateral ureteral catheterization and, once it is accomplished, the difficulty in properly wedging the catheters so that no urine escapes.

With newer techniques, particularly the refinement of rapid sequence IVP as a screening test, the Howard test is seldom performed because of the danger of introducing bacteria.

Radioactive renogram

This is a procedure in which radioactive material is injected intravenously. Special radiation detectors are placed over the kidneys for scanning.

Initially, this test was valued as a diagnostic tool in the evaluation of hypertension, particularly unilateral vascular renal hypertension. However, at the present time, the timed sequence IVP is the preferred screening test.

LABORATORY TESTS IN THE CLINICAL SETTING
Diseases affecting glomerular functional structural status
Acute glomerulonephritis

Acute glomerulonephritis is an acute inflammation that typically involves the glomerulus, although some minor changes are noted in the tubules.

Laboratory tests. Typical characteristic urine findings are mild to moderate proteinuria, hematuria, RBC casts, granular casts, and, depending on the diffuseness and extent of involvement, blood urea nitrogen retention indicating significant diminution of glomerular function.

Differential diagnosis. Previously glomerulonephritis was immediately equated with poststreptococcal nephritis. However, many other diseases are known to have renal involvement with the typical picture of glomerulonephritis. Thus, in the following discussion the other diseases will be mentioned and a differential diagnosis discussed.

Streptococcal pharyngitis or tonsillitis. This is the most common cause of acute glomerulonephritis. Therefore, if a patient presents for the first time with the urinary findings described above, a throat culture and a culture from any possible infected skin surface should be taken immediately because in a few situations, streptococcal infections can be initiated elsewhere than in the throat or tonsils. In addition to the urine findings the antistreptolysin-O titer will be elevated in approximately 75% of the cases. In the majority of cases involving a history of streptococcal pharyngitis and urine showing hematuria, albuminuria, RBCs, and protein casts, the diagnosis is quite simple. However, in more obscure cases the following diseases can be manifested as glomerulonephritis.

Systemic lupus erythematosus (SLE). Usually nephritis caused by systemic lupus erythematosus is not difficult to diagnose, especially in an established case. However, if the cause of the glomerulonephritis is still not established the serum level of antinuclear antibodies should be determined (see p. 181). The serum complement level is also important in evaluating the course of the renal involvement in SLE. A drop in serum complement level sometimes precedes the clinical appearance of lupus glomerulonephritis by about two weeks. Thus, serial and intermediate evaluation of the complement level in an established case of SLE helps significantly in the management of the case.

Serum sickness nephritis should also be checked in the differential diagnosis of patients with acute glomerulonephritis, as should Goodpasture's syndrome, in which glomerulonephritis is associated with pulmonary infiltration, hemoptysis, and arthritis. Other conditions associated with acute glomerulonephritis are subacute bacterial endocarditis, certain respiratory infections that can cause focal glomerulonephritis, hereditary nephritis, and nephritis associated with malignant hypertension.

The immune complex diseases as a cause of glomerulonephritis. Recently there has been a tendency to refer to the glomerulonephritides of various etiologies as the "immune complex diseases" (see p. 181). This includes all of the glomerulonephritides mentioned above as well as several other entities that are associated with renal involvement, such as the positive Australia antigen serum hepatitis (see p. 140) and Goodpasture's syndrome, all of which, though different, seem to have one common denominator—the deposition of immune complex particles on the basement membrane of blood vessels in many organs, including the glomeruli.

Chronic glomerulonephritis

Any of the processes mentioned above as a cause of acute glomerulonephritis eventually either heal completely or go into remissions and exacerbations, which are very similar to those found in acute glomerulonephritis.

Diagnostic laboratory tests. Persistent hematuria or proteinuria should lead the examiner to suspect latent chronic glomerulonephritis.

Differential diagnosis. When chronic glomerulonephritis progresses to end-stage kidney disease where there is persistent azotemia and elevated creatinine levels, it is sometimes impossible to differentiate among the following conditions: the chronic stage of acute glomerulonephritis, end-stage pyelonephritis, and end-stage nephrosclerosis.

Nephrotic syndrome

The disease state associated with massive proteinuria is the nephrotic syndrome. Protein appears in the urine because of significant alteration of the permeability of the glomerulus. There is usually also involvement of the tubules, allowing the marked leakage and excretion of protein and albumin.

Diagnostic laboratory tests. The diagnosis of nephrotic syndrome is made when a twenty four-hour urine specimen contains 3 gm or more of protein, which is usually found to be the albumin fraction of the serum proteins.

In addition to the massive proteinuria, the patient has an elevated cholesterol and hyperaldosteronemia with sodium and water retention and edema.

Differential diagnosis. More than fifty specific disease entities are characterized by the nephrotic syndrome in one stage of the disease. The more common ones include the following:
1. Nephrotic syndrome stage of acute glomerulonephritis, usually acute post-streptococcal, or any of the other acute glomerulonephritides
2. Metabolic causes such as diabetic nephropathy or amyloid kidney disease
3. Systemic disease such as collagenovascular disease and certain malignancies (multiple myeloma)
4. Circulatory disease such as renal vein thrombosis or right-sided congestive heart failure
5. Nephrotoxins such as heavy metals and lead poisoning
6. Certain allergens, drugs, infections, and miscellaneous entities

Diseases affecting tubular functional structural status
Acute tubular necrosis

This disease, also known as lower nephron nephrosis, is usually secondary to renal circulatory impairment and destruction of the renal tubules. There is also involvement of the glomeruli. However, the main pathology is at the tubular level.

Since acute tubular necrosis is reversible if properly managed and treated, it is important to make the correct diagnosis. The condition usually follows a state of shock, be it cardiogenic, toxic, or bacteremic, and it is usually the result of impaired circulation to the tubules.

Laboratory tests. Initially, the urine has a low specific gravity. Severe oliguria and anuria are the characteristic findings, with gradual elevation of blood urea nitrogen and creatinine.

If successfully treated, the patient experiences a polyuric phase in which are voided tremendous amounts of urine having a fixed specific gravity, while the BUN and creatinine may still be rising. At this stage, maintaining the electrolyte balance becomes very important for the management of the disease.

Differential diagnosis. When oliguria and anuria are present, the possibility of obstructive uropathy, a correctable condition, must always be considered.

Polyuric states

Differential diagnosis. When polyuria exists, the following possibilities should be considered. The polyuric phase of acute tubular necrosis has already been mentioned.

Diabetes insipidus. This is not a renal disease, but because of the absence of ADH, which is responsible for the reabsorption of water from the distal tubules, there is a massive polyuria sometimes approaching fifteen to twenty liters a day. Although ADH is absent, the renal response to ADH is normal. An injection of ADH corrects the polyuria of diabetes insipidus, whereas polyuria secondary to renal tubular disease does not respond to ADH.

Recently, it has been found that chlorpropamide (Diabinese) has an action similar to ADH on the distal tubular cells and partially corrects the polyuria of diabetes insipidus. This is helpful in the differential diagnosis of diabetes insipidus versus renal tubular disease.

Renal tubular diseases. This group of diseases is also associated with polyuria because of the impairment of the reabsorption of water and electrolytes. Polyuric states can, therefore, be seen in hypercalcemic nephropathy, hypokalemic nephropathy, and in certain kinds of renal tubular acidosis of hereditary conditions.

Renal tubular disease also is usually associated with abnormal excretion of amino acids, such as cystinuria and the De-Fanconi syndrome.

Analgesic nephropathy. This disease simulates renal tubular acidosis and is characterized by polyuria and azotemia with a more or less fixed specific gravity. Again, this is because of the tubular involvement secondary to the analgesics, which impair absorption. The most common of the analgesic nephropathies is the phenacetin nephropathy.

Congenital anomalies

From a therapeutic point of view, recognition of the congenital anomalies is important because of the predisposition of patients with these conditions to repeated urinary tract infection.

Laboratory tests. The patient should be checked frequently with urine culture, which will identify the infecting organism.

Differential diagnosis. Horseshoe kidney and polycystic kidney are among the congenital entities. Polycystic kidney disease also enters into the differential diagnosis of hypertension and is associated with a certain percentage of berry aneurysms and intracranial hemorrhage.

Renal vascular hypertension

The hypertension associated with renal vascular disease may be the result of a pathologic state at the level of the major renal vessels (obstructive vascular disease) or at the level of the smaller arteries and arterioles (nephrosclerosis). The pathologic finding of nephrosclerosis in an elderly person's kidney is not too uncommon and is found in generalized atherosclerosis. Besides the general atherosclerotic process involving the smaller arteries, there are several curious conditions in which there is only unilateral or bilateral involvement of the renal artery. Significant narrowing of these arteries can occur and result from either fibromuscular hyperplasia, which is common in females between 35 and 45 years of age, or an atherosclerotic plaque that narrows the renal artery to such a degree that an appreciable pressure gradient is created on either side of the obstruction. This situation triggers a hormone system called the renin-angiotensin system, which causes hypertension by the mechanism described on p. 110. The hypertension thus produced eventually affects the kidneys further by causing more nephrosclerotic changes in the renal arteries thus establishing a self-perpetuating cycle. It is imperative that patients with this disease be identified, particularly those in the younger age group for whom surgical correction of the disease is possible.

Laboratory tests

Renal vascular hypertension may manifest with minor, nonspecific urinary findings such as a few red blood cells with some RBC casts and a slight diminution of glomerular filtration rate (creatinine clearance).

Differential diagnosis

The tests employed for differentiating renal vascular hypertension from other hypertensions, as well as for presurgical evaluation, are listed below in the order of their importance and yield. Because of the technical difficulties and interpretation problems attendant to split renal function tests, they are being done less often.

1. Timed (rapid) sequence IVP should be done in the absence of significant BUN elevation. Renal artery stenosis is suspected if the dye appears in one kidney five or ten minutes after the other kidney. The IVP is also helpful in evaluating the kidney size, which is another parameter of renal vascular hypertension, the small kidney having the compromised vascular supply.
2. Assessment of peripheral blood renin levels, and, if possible, independent measurement of the the renin secretory rate from each renal vein, which is accomplished by selectively catheterizing the renal veins.
3. Renal arteriography ultimately establishes the diagnosis. However, this test should not be done until the patient has been screened with rapid sequence IVP.
4. The Howard test (split renal function test) is seldom performed.

Diseases associated with pure hematuria

Pure hematuria usually indicates a disease process below the nephron, which can be anywhere from the collecting ducts to the bladder. In this situation there are usually no RBC casts and the microscopic examination of the urine shows gross RBCs.

Painless hematuria

If there is no pain associated with the hematuria the examiner should suspect renal tumors, renal tuberculosis, or inflammatory or malignant disease involving the structures below the nephron, that is, the collecting ducts, kidney pelvis, ureters, or bladder.

Painful hematuria

Nephrolithiasis is usually painful, particularly when obstructing the urinary tract or while moving in the ureters. However, a big staghorn calculus located in the pelvis of the kidney may be asymptomatic and a cause of intermitent pure hematuria.

Pure pyuria and bacteruria

In an acute case of fever, chills, and pyuria the diagnosis is acute pyelonephritis. This usually affects the renal parenchyma as well as the tubules and the collecting ducts in the renal pelvis, and eventually the bladder. Under such circumstances it is imperative that a urine culture be obtained to identify the organism. The most common organism in an otherwise uncomplicated case is *E. coli.*

When there are repeated episodes of acute pyelonephritis, the examiner should investigate the kidney for any possible correctable structural conditions that may predispose to repeated pyelonephritis. Unless this is done and the condition is corrected, the patient may develop chronic pyelonephritis. Under such circumstances an IV pyelogram and an excretory cystourogram are usually done to rule out reflux at the cystourethral junction. Any indication of chronicity warrants a thorough investigation of the genitrourinary tract for partial obstructive uropathy.

CHAPTER 7

Diagnostic tests for gastrointestinal disorders

ANATOMY AND PHYSIOLOGY

The gastrointestinal (GI) system is unique both anatomically and functionally. Anatomically it begins in the oral cavity and ends in the anal orifice. Accessory organs, either located in the main digestive tract or opening into it, include the salivary glands, teeth, liver, gallbladder, pancreas, and appendix as illustrated in Fig. 7-1.

The digestive system forms a tube all the way through the ventral cavities of the body. It is, therefore, possible with fiberoptic scopes to directly visualize most of the GI tract. In addition to this, the laboratory studies can be directed toward the GI functions: propelling the nutritional items from the oral cavity to the different parts of the digestive tract and, breaking down these nutritional items into absorbable units by secreting chemical juices.

The anatomy and physiology of the accessory organs will be discussed separately.

LABORATORY TESTS FOR GASTROINTESTINAL DISEASES

Since a study of the gastrointestinal tract involves not only the main digestive tract, but the accessory organs as well, the diagnostic laboratory tests are covered under each division of the digestive tract and each accessory organ. A few general observations follow.

Direct visualization

The fiberoptic scope directly visualizes previously inaccessible structures and performs the usual endoscopic procedures easier and with less hazard and discomfort to the patient.

The fiberoptic scope consists of a rope of very thin, flexible, transparent fibers through which light can be bent around corners, taken into tiny crevices, and slid through narrow slits. The light from a light source is transmitted down some of the fibers; from the illuminated area the light is then reflected back up the remaining fibers to produce an image. The modern endoscope has a tip deflection of 180 degrees

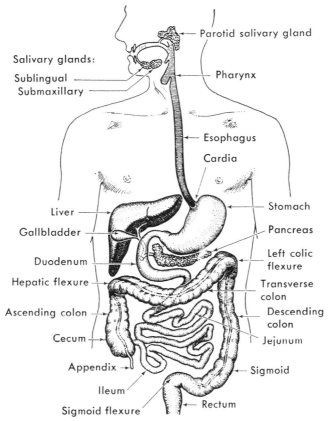

Fig. 7-1. The gastrointestinal system and accessory organs. (From Schottelius, B. A., and Schottelius, D. D.: Textbook of physiology, ed. 17, St. Louis, 1973, The C. V. Mosby Co.)

and is equipped with channels to permit the passage of biopsy forceps, cytology brushes, irrigating or injecting cannulas, snares, and cautery.

Upper gastrointestinal endoscopy permits visualization of all portions of the esophagus, stomach, and duodenum (panendoscopy). Direct visualization of the entire colonic mucosa is now possible with the fiberoptic colonoscope. Proctosigmoidoscopy and rectal examination are still the procedures most likely to detect the site and source of lower gastrointestinal bleeding.

Radiologic examination

Radiologic examination involves the introduction of a contrast medium into the gastrointestinal tract (barium enema, barium swallow, oral cholecystography) or into the circulatory system (selective angiography) so that the outline of the structures and pathologic anomalies can be observed on x-ray film.

If a thorough study of the GI tract is necessary the oral cholecystogram should be performed first, followed by the barium enema and then the upper GI series.

The dangers of introducing barium into the GI tract should be taken into consideration as well as the dangers of the preparation for the procedure. The use of strong cathartics in the presence of obstructing lesions of the colon or small intestine or in the presence of active ulcerative colitis may be hazardous or life-threatening. The barium may aggravate acute ulcerative colitis or cause a partial obstruction to become complete.

A major disadvantage of contrast barium studies in the presence of gastrointestinal bleeding is the inability to associate an observed lesion with the bleeding site. If lesions are multiple, then the bleeding site should be established by panendoscopy.

Motility and pressure studies

Manometric studies are particularly valuable in evaluating esophageal function. A manometer is an instrument used to measure the pressure of liquids or gases. Abnormal pressures and abnormal motilities can be delineated when a manometric catheter is advanced through the oral cavity toward the cervical esophagus and combined with barium swallow and x-ray films.

THE ESOPHAGUS
Anatomy and physiology

The esophagus (Fig. 7-1) extends from the pharynx to the stomach. It is a collapsible tube about 10 inches long through which the bolus of food is propelled after having been swallowed. An initial peristaltic wave originates in the pharynx and secondary peristaltic waves originate in the esophagus if food still remains there. The lower end of the esophagus acts as a physiologic sphincter to prevent the reflux of food from the stomach. This is sometimes referred to as the cardiac sphincter because of its relationship to the cardia of the stomach.

Laboratory tests
Bernstein test

The Bernstein test demonstrates reflux esophagitis. Hydrochloric acid (HCl) 0.1% is started as a drip into the esophagus after normal saline has first been used. Spontaneous symptoms produced in the patient within one half hour after the HCl drip starts are indicative of esophagitis.

In order to definitely verify whether the HCl is causing the esophageal symptoms, The saline drip can be used as the control. If the patient has no symptoms when again given the saline but develops typical symptoms of esophagitis when the HCl drip is reinstated, reflux esophagitis is indicated.

Test for esophageal acidity

In addition to reflux esophagitis, the acidity of the esophagus can also be demonstrated. After the HCl drip is instituted as described above, the pH of the esophagus will remain in the range of above five or six if the sphincter at the junction of the esophagus and the stomach is competent. However, if there is a reflux, the pH will fall intermittently to 1.5 or two, indicating free reflux of acid from the stomach to the lower esophagus.

Laboratory tests in the clinical setting
Esophagitis

The most common disease entity affecting esophageal function is probably esophagitis. This disease is usually secondary to the irritating effect of reflux of gastric juice from the stomach into the lower part of the esophagus.

Laboratory tests. The most common laboratory tests employed in the diagnosis of reflux esophagitis are radiologic studies demonstrating reflux of a contrast material, the Bernstein test, and the demonstration of esophageal acidity.

Differential diagnosis. In reflux esophagitis a radiologic diagnosis of hiatal hernia is frequently made. However, The mere demonstration of hiatal hernia is not necessarily an indication that reflux exists; nor does it necessarily indicate that the symptoms produced are a result of the hiatal hernia causing the reflux. Many hiatal hernias are found in asymptomatic patients, and though an associated reflux has been shown to cause symptoms of esophagitis, hiatal hernia as a cause of esophagitis should be questioned. If there are chronic symptoms of recurrent esophagitis causing this failure and motility disturbance this can be demonstrated radiologicaly or cineradiographically. However, occasionally esophagoscopy and biopsy are important since not all chronic esophagitis is due to chronic reflux esophagitis. Sometimes it may be due to other diseases, such as cancer and scleroderma, thus, making esophageal biopsy with an esophagoscope mandatory.

Diffuse esophageal spasm

Diffuse esophageal spasm is probably the second most common of the esophageal diseases. It is a disorder of esophageal motility of various etiologies including reflux esophagitis.

Laboratory tests. The diagnosis is best made radiologicaly with a cine-esophagogram that shows the disturbed segmental contractions without a peristaltic wave in the distal esophagus. This disorder can also be confirmed with manometric pressure studies of the different parts of the esophagus.

Differential diagnosis. Diffuse esophageal spasm is commonly associated with aging (presbyesophagus), ganglion degeneration (seen in the early stages of achalasia), mucosal irritation (most likely secondary to gastroesophageal reflux), obstruction of the cardia, and neuromuscular disorders (diabetic neuropathy and amyotrophic lateral sclerosis). Sometimes it may simply be called idiopathic.

Achalasia

Achalasia is a motor disorder, the symptoms of which appear to reflect impaired cholinergic innervation of the esophagus.

Laboratory tests. The diagnosis is made with radiologic contrast studies showing the abnormal esophageal motor function with a characteristic beaklike narrowing of the distal esophageal segment.

Differential diagnosis. Occasionally diffuse esophageal spasm may, over the years, evolve into achalasia. Sometimes, in the differential diagnosis, carcinoma of the lower esophagus becomes a problem and esophagoscopic study with biopsy is most helpful. Other esophageal problems considered in the differential diagnosis include the following.

Scleroderma (progressive systemic sclerosis) involves the esophagus 80% of the time and is characterized by the loss of esophageal peristalsis.

Dermatomyositis is characterized by oral pharangeal dysphagia with difficulty in propelling the bolus from the mouth to the esophagus.

Neurologic conditions may possibly affect deglutition. One must be aware of the possibility of myasthenia gravis in deglutition problems. Edrophonium chloride (Tensilon) can be used for diagnostic testing. If the muscular weakness is caused by myasthenia gravis, the edrophonium injection will produce prompt relief.

The esophagus may rupture spontaneously, sometimes in previously healthy individuals. Usually x-ray films will show free air in the mediastinum with resultant mediastinal crunch and subcutaneous emphysema. Hydropneumothorax secondary to digestion of the mediastinal pleura by gastric acid may be present, and, occasionally, severe hemorrhage associated with vertical laceration of the gastroesophageal junction (Mallory-Weiss syndrome).

Plummer-Vinson syndrome consists of dysphagia associated with iron deficiency anemia and usually is found in elderly females.

THE STOMACH
Anatomy and physiology

The stomach and its relationship to the rest of the digestive tract, the liver, and the pancreas is illustrated in Fig. 7-1. After the food enters the stomach it is stored, mixed with gastric juice, and then slowly emptied into the small intestine through the pyloric sphincter.

The gastric juice is secreted by the gastric glands in the walls of the stomach. Gastric juice is normally clear, pale yellow and of high acidity with a pH of about 1.0. It is 97% to 99% water, 0.2% to 0.5% HCl, with the remainder consisting of mucin, inorganic salts, digestive enzymes (pepsin and rennin), and a lipase.

Stimulation of gastric juice secretion is initiated by psychic factors that activate the vagus nerve. Vagal impulses directly stimulate the parietal cells to secrete acid and the mucosa to secrete a hormone, *gastrin*, which is absorbed into the blood and carried back to the stomach to stimulate gastric secretion. *Histamine*, which is derived from an amino acid, also is a potent stimulus to gastric secretion.

Laboratory tests for gastric acid analysis

Gastric acid studies are done for the following indications:
1. To determine whether the patient is able to secrete acid. This is done to establish

the differential diagnosis of gastric ulcer. The inability to secrete acid practically rules out a benign gastric ulcer.

2. To determine how much acid the patient secretes. This is indicated in rare conditions in which the clinical diagnosis strongly suggests peptic ulcer disease with an equivocal upper GI series. A high basal secretion (10 mEq or more) is practically diagnostic of active peptic ulcer disease.

3. To determine the type of surgery necessary. In hypersecretors, there is increased risk of stomal ulcer following ordinary gastric resection without vagotomy. If the patient is still having symptoms after a vagotomy for peptic ulcer, the completeness of the vagotomy should be ascertained by a Hollander test, which is explained below.

Basal secretion

Determination of basal secretion is performed to ascertain how much acid the patient secretes without stimulation to do so. The patient is intubated under fluoroscopic visualization. The gastric contents are then aspirated continuously for two hours, with the aspirate titrated at half-hour intervals. A secretion of 6 mEq or more per hour is indicative of hypersecretion. A secretion of 15 mEq or more should lead one to suspect a hormonal abnormality affecting the parietal cells.

NORMAL BASAL ACID OUTPUT (BAO)

0-6 mEq/hr

Histalog gastric analysis

Since the capacity of the gastric cells to secrete may not, on a particular occasion, be significant in the basal state, betazole hydrochloride (Histalog) may be injected. With this stimulus a secretion in excess of 50 mEq/hr indicates hypersecretion.

Hollander test

This test is performed in order to determine whether a vagotomy has been complete or not. The patient is given an injection of insulin to produce hypoglycemia. The hypoglycemia should be 50% of fasting blood sugar. If the gastric secretion in any postinsulin hour (two hours) exceeds that of the higher of the two basal hours, (pre-insulin fasting stage, two determinations) the vagotomy is incomplete. The patient should have a preoperative Hollander test in order to help interpret this later test.

Gastric analysis using calcium infusion

The differential diagnosis between hypersecretory states with and without inappropriate gastrin production (Zollinger-Ellison syndrome) can be made by performing the gastric analysis while the patient is receiving calcium infusion. Serum gastrin levels are measured in the basal state and again during calcium infusion. If the secretion of gastric acid approaches maximal levels and the serum gastrin levels rise appreciably with the calcium infusion, ectopic gastrin production, such as is seen in Zollinger-Ellison syndrome, is suspected.

Gastric analysis using secretin

This is another test performed to differentiate the Zollinger-Ellison syndrome from hypersecretory states without inappropriate secretion of gastrin. Secretin is given intravenously and should cause a decrease in acid secretion. However, with Zollinger-Ellison syndrome the acid secretion is increased to maximum Histalog levels and the serum gastrin rises.

Laboratory tests in the clinical setting
Castritis

The most common disorder of the stomach is probably superficial gastritis secondary to ingestion of irritants such as aspirin and/or alcohol.

Laboratory tests. The diagnosis of gastritis is usually made by gastroscopy, since superficial gastritis may not be visualized by barium studies. However, the acute inflammatory edematous mucosa can easily be seen with a gastroscope.

Gastric ulcer disease

Gastric ulcer disease is probably less common than gastritis.

Laboratory tests. The diagnosis depends on *radiologic* and *gastroscopic examination*. The combination of these two tests brings the diagnostic accuracy up to approximately 90% or 95%.

Differential diagnosis. In differentiating between benign and malignant gastric ulcer, radiologic examination of the stomach is probably the most important diagnostic aid. However, during a gastroscopic procedure, a mucosal biopsy can be performed in suspected cases of carcinoma.

Cytologic examination of the gastric juice depends on the expertise of the pathologist and the accuracy varies from 30% to 80%.

Gastric acid examination is of some help. If true histamine-fast achlorhydria is present, then there is no good, reassuring way of ruling out the diagnosis of carcinoma. However, the presence of acid does not necessarily rule out carcinoma either.

If malignancy is not established with the above tests, strict medical therapy should be initiated. The radiologic examination should then be repeated between the second and third week of intensive medical therapy. If there is a reduction of the ulcer size by 50% or more then the lesion is probably benign and the medical regime should be continued for two or three more weeks until there is complete healing. The gastric studies should then be repeated.

Duodenal peptic ulcer

Laboratory tests. *X-ray contrast barium study* is the most definitive diagnostic step in confirming the presence of duodenal ulcer. The demonstration of a crater on the films is the main characteristic of peptic ulcer disease.

Differential diagnosis. *Gastric juice analysis* is usually not important in ordinary ulcer disease, with two possible exceptions: Histamine-fast achlorhydria rules out peptic ulcer disease. In malignant and severe peptic ulcer disease the gastric acid secretion rate may be important particularly in a diagnosis of Zollinger-Ellison syndrome, which is a peptic ulceration associated with a nonbeta cell islet tumor of the pancreas that releases excessive gastrin resulting in profound gastric hypersecretion.

Stomal or gastrojejunal ulceration

A radiographic diagnosis of stomal ulcer is extremely difficult because of the altered anatomy and because two thirds to three fourths of stomal ulcers cannot be visualized radiographically. However, the stoma and the ulceration can be visualized quite easily through a gastroscope.

Zollinger-Ellison syndrome

The Zollinger-Ellison syndrome is characterized by profound gastric hypersecretion that causes a typical and severe malignant peptic ulceration.

Laboratory tests. When there is a minimum increase in the maximum output of acid in response to further stimulation by histamine, Zollinger-Ellison syndrome may be present. A careful determination of the one hour basal acid output coupled with the maximum histamine stimulation provides as much information as is necessary for this diagnosis.

Complications of peptic ulcer

Hemorrhage. In upper GI hemorrhage it is essential to document the site of bleeding. Thus, a vigorous, aggressive diagnostic approach is recommended. It is negligent to assume that the bleeding is from esophageal varices when the patient has cirrhosis of the liver. The bleeding might be a result of a gastric ulcer or a duodenal ulcer.

Laboratory tests. Intubation of the stomach should be performed on every patient with GI bleeding. In order to locate the lesion precisely, gentle aspiration through the intestinal tube should be carried out while the tube is being passed. This should be done at 20 to 30 minute intervals, the aspirate being observed for blood. If blood is noted, barium is given and the area is studied.

If upper GI bleeding is massive, a large gastric tube should be introduced, the clots removed, and the area irrigated with iced saline. An emergency GI series can then be performed.

Perforation. Of patients with perforated ulcers, 85% have free air under the diaphragm that can be detected by x-ray examination of the abdomen with the patient in a reclining and an upright position. It should be noted, however, that the absence of free air under the diaphragm does not necessarily rule out perforation.

An elevated serum amylase correlating with the clinical picture is extremely suggestive of perforation.

Occasionally, in equivocal cases, the perforation may be identified through the use of water-soluble contrast material (Gastrografin).

Gastric outlet obstruction. Obstruction of the outlet of the stomach is usually due to active ulceration and edema.

Laboratory tests. X-ray films reveal a huge, dilated stomach, often occupying most of the abdomen.

Differential diagnosis. A course of judicious medical treatment with decompression and continuous suction with replacement of electrolytes differentiates between organic obstruction and inflammatory edema. Barium studies should not be done until the stomach has been decompressed and cleansed, since it is difficult or impossible to accurately assess the cause of the obstruction under these circumstances.

THE SMALL INTESTINE
Anatomy and physiology

The small intestine is a tube approximately one inch in diameter and twenty feet in length. It begins at the pyloric end of the stomach (duodenum), which can be seen in Fig. 7-1 in the shape of a C around the pancreas. The jejunum and ileum constitute the rest of the small bowel.

The chyme is propelled through the small bowel by segmentation contractions and peristalsis, and digestion is completed by the action of the intestinal juice. The end products of digestion are then absorbed into the blood and lymph.

Laboratory tests for malabsorption syndromes
Fecal fat content

This is the best screening test for overall malabsorption syndrome. The total twenty-four-hour fecal fat should be less than 6 gm per twenty-four hours. If it is more than 6, malabsorption is indicated. However, this does not differentiate between pancreatic and intestinal intrinsic malabsorption.

Serum carotenes and prothrombin time

Since absorption of the fat-soluble vitamins is impaired in fat malabsorptive states, serum carotene levels and prothrombin time are diminished. The abnormal bleeding time results from vitamin K deficiency.

D-xylose absorption

This is a useful test and usually indicates intrinsic intestinal disease problems when it is positive. D-xylose is normally not metabolized and is absorbed intact. Intrinsic intestinal disease, particularly in the proximal intestine, is reflected by diminished D-xylose absorption.

Gastrointestinal x-ray films

Radiographic films are extremely helpful in providing clues of gastroileostomy, scleroderma, Zollinger-Ellison syndrome, ulcerative colitis, and intestinal fistulas as possible causes of malabsorption.

Small intestinal biopsy

Small intestinal biopsy is of diagnostic value in the following conditions: agammaglobulinemia, Whipple's disease, celiac sprue, and abetalipoproteinemia. Biopsy may also be of value in the diagnosis of intestinal lymphoma, amyloidosis, eosinophilic enteritis, regional enteritis, intestinal lymphangiectasis, systemic mastocytosis, and parasitic infestations.

This test is not diagnostic although it may be abnormal in systemic scleroderma, acute radiation enteritis, tropical sprue, vitamin B_{12} deficiency, bacterial overgrowth syndromes, and folate deficiency.

Secretin test

The secretin test is probably the most important test in differentiating between malabsorption secondary to pancreatic disease and intrinsic intestinal disease. Secretin is a hormone that stimulates the pancreatic production of a thin, watery fluid high in bicarbonate content but low in enzyme content. After the passage of a double lumen tube for separate gastric and duodenal aspiration, secretin is given intravenously. The gastric and duodenal contents are collected separately with the latter being measured for volume, bicarbonate content, and amylase activity. A volume of less than 1.5 ml/kg body weight per thirty minutes, or a bicarbonate concentration less than 70 mEq/l indicates subnormal pancreatic function. Cytologic examination of the aspirate may be helpful in the diagnosis of carcinoma.

Flat film of the abdomen

In addition to the secretin test, a flat film of the abdomen that visualizes pancreatic calcification is extremely helpful in differentiating chronic pancreatitis from intrinsic intestinal disease as a possible cause of steatorrhea and malabsorption.

Celiac angiogram

The celiac angiogram often delineates a pancreatic tumor or a pancreatic cyst secondary to acute pancreatitis as the cause of malabsorption.

Trioleic and oleic absorption tests

Because of the technical difficulties and inaccuracies, the trioleic and oleic absorption tests, which differentiate between pancreatic and intrinsic bowel malabsorption, are of very limited value and seldom used for differential diagnosis purposes at the present time.

Schilling test for vitamin B_{12} absorption

This test is of value in differentiating between an intrinsic factor deficiency and an absorption problem in the distal ilium, where vitamin B_{12} is primarily absorbed.

There are two factors necessary for the formation of red blood cells: the extrinsic factor (vitamin B_{12}), which is found in meat, eggs, milk, and the like, and the intrinsic factor, which is produced by the gastric mucosa. The function of the intrinsic factor is to assure the absorption of vitamin B_{12}.

The Schilling test is performed by first giving the patient oral radioactive vitamin B_{12}. Two hours later a massive nonradioactive parenteral dose is given. About one third of the absorbed vitamin should appear in the urine; therefore, the presence of little or no radioactivity in the urine indicates gastrointestinal malabsorption. If there is absorption, ilial disease is ruled out as a cause of malabsorption, and since the vitamin was given without the intrinsic factor, pernicious anemia is also ruled out.

The same procedure is again followed with the addition of the intrinsic factor to the oral vitamin B_{12}. Nonabsorption of the vitamin B_{12} without the intrinsic factor, but absorption of it when the intrinsic factor is added is diagnostic of pernicious anemia.

Occasionally, a patient may not absorb vitamin B_{12} with or without the intrinsic factor because of excessive bacterial invasion such as would occur in the blind loop syndrome. In this case, the results of the Schilling test return to normal after a course of antibiotic therapy.

Laboratory tests in the clinical setting

Malabsorption syndrome

The malabsorption syndrome will be best understood after some physiological considerations relative to digestion and absorption are reviewed briefly.

The digestive processes initiated in the stomach are continued in the upper small intestine mainly by the action of pancreatic enzymes. These digestive processes result in the breakdown of carbohydrates to monosaccharides and disaccharides, proteins to peptides and amino acids, and fats to monoglycerides and fatty acids. In this form the nutrients are absorbed across the intestinal cell into the capillaries and then into the general circulation through the portal system or into the intestinal lymphatics through the lacteals. The motility of the small intestine and its total surface area are factors in its absorptive capabilities, as are adequate pancreatic and biliary secretions. Thus, malabsorption syndromes are divided into two major categories: those due to intrinsic small intestinal wall disease with normal digestion but abnormal absorption because of intrinsic lesions of the bowel wall and those due to digestive problems related to pancreatic insufficiency or bile acid secretory problems causing delayed or inadequate absorption.

The differential diagnosis is made by means of the tests for malabsorption syndrome, previously described.

Mesenteric arterial insufficiency

The mesenteric arteries supply the splanchnic area. Atherosclerotic or other degenerative changes in these arteries or the celiac axis can produce pain that is steady and agonizing. Mucosal changes and mural deterioration lead to malabsorption, causing weight loss and symptoms of malabsorption.

Vascular insufficiency in elderly patients may contribute significantly to malabsorption. The syndrome in these patients may be at the subclinical level and be undetected if not looked for particularly.

To evaluate the vascular integrity of the GI tract, celiac angiogram and superior and inferior mesenteric angiograms are quite helpful in selected and individualized cases.

Inflammatory intestinal disease (regional enteritis)

Initial suspicion of this disease comes from chronic intermittent diarrhea, crampy abdominal pain, joint pains, and abdominal masses revealed by the physical examination. Perianal ulceration and stricture is quite common.

Laboratory tests. Nonspecific laboratory findings are leukocytosis, blood loss, anemia, undernutrition, hypoalbuminemia, hypocalcemia, hypokalemia, elevated sedimentation rate, elevated serum alkaline phosphatase level, hypoprothrombinemia, and macrocytic anemia.

The radiologic picture along with the clinical suspicion usually establishes the diagnosis. It is definitely established histologically. Fistulous tracts are common, particularly in the ileocecal region, and are virtually pathognomonic.

In the operating room, biopsies of the small intestine and lymph nodes provide adequate bases for microscopic diagnosis and rule out tuberculosis, various lymphomas, sarcoidosis, and fungous diseases.

Acute intestinal obstruction

Laboratory tests. Flat films of the abdomen are the most important single examination in suspected cases of intestinal obstruction. From the type of lumen pattern, the level of obstruction can more or less be determined. If the symptoms are acute and the obstruction is suspected to be low in the intestine, barium should not be given orally. However, if the obstruction is thought to be in the colon, then a carefully administered barium enema may demonstrate the obstructive lesion.

The other laboratory findings of intestinal obstruction are nonspecific inflammatory findings such as leukocytosis, the distention of the acute abdomen, lactic dehydrogenase elevation, and grossly bloody stools when a large area of the small intestine is being strangulated.

THE COLON
Anatomy and physiology

The large intestine is approximately five or six feet in length and two and a half inches in diameter. It begins at the cecum and proceeds in turn as the ascending colon, transverse colon, descending colon, sigmoid colon, rectum, and anal canal (Fig. 7-1). The functions of the colon are the absorption of water and electrolytes from the chyme and the storage and elimination of waste products of digestion.

Laboratory tests
Radiologic examination

Radiologic examination of the colon is a most important diagnostic tool. It should be noted, however that acutely ill patients do not tolerate well the necessary preparation for barium enema. If the patient is not acutely ill a diagnosis can be determined by a simple barium enema or by air contrast barium enema, which is even more diagnostic. The barium enema is employed for the possible diagnosis of malignancies, benign growth, diverticular disease, inflammatory disease of the GI tract such as ulcerative colitis and regional enteritis, and nonspecific granulomatous disease such as inflammatory disease that cannot be classified. Also included in this list are the bacterial granulomatous diseases such as tuberculous enteritis and colitis or amebic colitis.

In some of the conditions mentioned above the specific diagnosis can be made fairly well by the barium enema alone. However, often more direct visual examination and biopsy are necessary. Therefore, the second most important test in the examination of the colon is sigmoidoscopy.

Sigmoidoscopy

This test is used for two major reasons. The lower 15 to 18 cm of the colon is difficult to visualize radiologically, particularly the sigmoid region, but is easily seen through a sigmoidoscope. The definitive diagnosis in certain conditions can be achieved through biopsy under direct visualization, which is possible with sigmoidoscopy. Ulceration is seen easily, and a biopsy is the determining factor in the differential diagnosis between ulcerative colitis and amebic colitis.

Colonoscopy

Recently, with the advent of the fiberoptic scopes, it has been possible to scope the whole colon. Colonoscopy, in experienced hands, is another direct visual means by which the colon can be examined and biopsy can be taken.

Rectal biopsy

This test is of significant importance in certain conditions such as amyloidosis and some parasitic diseases such as schistosomiasis and regional enteritis.

THE GALLBLADDER
Anatomy and physiology

The gallbladder is a pear-shaped sac lying on the underside of the liver. Bile is produced by the liver and enters the gallbladder by the hepatic and cystic ducts to be concentrated and stored until needed.

During digestion, the gallbladder contracts and rapidly supplies bile to the small intestine through the common bile duct (Fig. 7-2). This contraction of the gallbladder and also the relaxation of the sphincter muscle is in response to a hormone (cholecystokinin) that is secreted by the intestine in the presence of meat and fats.

Laboratory tests
Oral cholecystography

With this most effective diagnostic test several pathologic entities can be described. They are as follows:
1. If a normal gallbladder with a few gallstones is visualized, the implication is

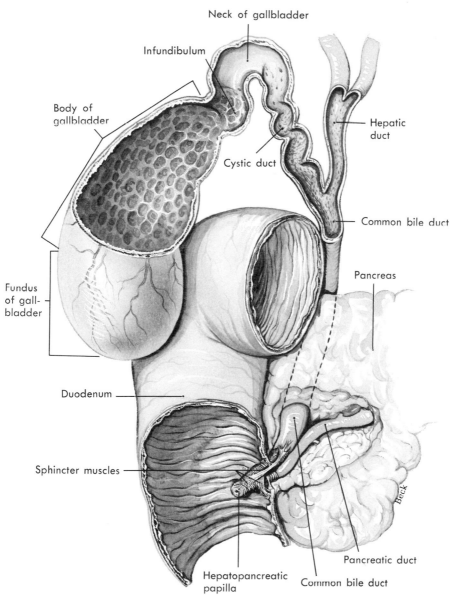

Neck of gallbladder

Infundibulum

Body of
gallbladder

Cystic duct

Hepatic
duct

Common bile duct

Pancreas

Fundus
of gall-
bladder

Duodenum

Sphincter muscles

Hepatopancreatic
papilla

Common bile duct

Pancreatic duct

Fig. 7-2. The gallbladder and its divisions: fundus, body, infundibulum, and neck. Obstruction of either the hepatic or common bile duct by stone or spasm blocks the exit of bile from the liver, where it is formed, and prevents bile from ejecting into the duodenum. (From Anthony, C. P., and Kolthoff, N. J.: Textbook of anatomy and physiology, ed. 9, St. Louis, 1975, The C. V. Mosby Co.)

that the patient's symptoms arise while the gallstones are passing through the gallbladder ducts.

2. If, after a second dose of contrast media, the gallbladder is still not visualized, and if there is no indication of a GI lesion by either poor absorption or rapid transit of the dye, one should then assume that the gallbladder is not concentrating the dye for excretion. This implies a chronically inflamed gallbladder, which most likely contains gravel-type gallstones. This has specific clinical implications for the patient.

3. If a solitary, large gallstone is visualized, the implication is that the gallbladder is functioning normally and probably is healthy, except for the stone, which probably will not cause symptoms since it is too large to be passed.

Intravenous cholecystography

Intravenous cholecystography eliminates the oral absorption factor in gallbladder disease, thus permitting certain visualization of the gallbladder if it is healthy and eliminating GI factors of absorption. There is also the additional advantage of being able to visualize the ducts slightly better than with oral cholecystography.

Therefore, if by oral cholecystography not all of the necessary information is obtained, particularly concerning the gallbladder duct, intravenous cholecystography may be an adjunct in the diagnosis and management of gallbladder problems.

Of course, both intravenous and oral cholecystography should be performed when the patient is free of jaundice. Otherwise, because of liver disease, the patient will not be able to metabolize and concentrate the dye in the gallbladder. Thus, when the situation is grave and the diagnosis must be made between obstructive jaundice and hepatocellular jaundice, *percutaneous cholangiography* can be utilized.

Percutaneous cholangiography

This test will differentiate major obstructive jaundice from hepatocellular jaundice. The procedure accomplished by inserting a needle into the liver and then into a dilated intrahepatic duct. Bile is then drained and dye is injected. The obstruction is thus visualized in 75% to 90% of cases.

Operative cholangiography

This procedure is carried out during surgery and involves the introduction of dye into the biliary tracts or gallbladder, followed by x-ray films. In this way it can be ascertained if the biliary tracts are free of pathology or stones.

Fiberoptic duodenoscopy

With this technique, the ampulla of Vater (Fig. 7-2) can be intubated under direct vision and dye can be injected with excellent results, giving further information in difficult cases.

Other tests

Currently, increasing use is being made of selective angiography of the celiac, superior mesenteric, and hepatic arteries for the purpose of visualizing the portal and hepatic circulation. However, these procedures are done only in highly specialized centers for the more complicated and difficult cases.

Hypotonic duodenography is also being used in the differential diagnosis of intraabdominal problems to differentiate between pancreatic tumors and pancreatitis.

THE LIVER
Anatomy and physiology

The liver is the largest gland and the major metabolic factory in the human body. It lies immediately under the diaphragm, occupying most of the right upper quadrant (Fig. 7-1). The liver is involved in protein synthesis and other metabolic functions, regulation of blood volume, immune mechanisms, formation and excretion of bile, and the detoxification and excretion of toxic elements. The function of the liver is also important in the synthesis, esterification, and excretion of cholesterol.

There are three major types of cell in the liver, the hepatocytes, the biliary epithelial cells, and the Kupffer cells. Most metabolic functions are carried out by the hepatocytes. The Kupffer cells belong to the reticuloendothelial system, and the biliary cells line the biliary system, the gall bladder, the bile ducts, and the canaliculi.

Physiologic basis for liver function tests

Bilirubin. This is the chief bile pigment in man. It originates in the reticuloendothelial cells of the liver and other reticuloendothelial cells, being formed by the breakdown of hemoglobin, and normally bound to albumin in the circulation. Bilirubin is then carried to the liver where it is conjugated with glucuronic acid. This *conjugated bilirubin* is more water soluble than the *free bilirubin,* and therefore passes more easily into the intestine with the bile. Once within the intestine, the bilirubin is reduced to *urobilinogen* by the action of intestinal bacteria. Some of this urobilinogen is absorbed into the circulation and is either excreted in the urine or reexcreted in the bile. The rest of the intestinal urobilinogen is excreted in the stool as *fecal urobilinogen.*

Jaundice. Excessive bilirubin in the blood escapes into the tissues, which turn yellow (jaundice). Jaundice shows best on the sclera. Its causes include the following:
1. More bilirubin is produced than the normal liver can excrete (hemolytic jaundice).
2. A damaged liver may not be able to excrete normal amounts of bilirubin (hepatic jaundice).
3. An obstruction of the excretory ducts prevents the excretion of bilirubin (obstructive jaundice).

Bile accumulates in the blood in all of these conditions and at certain concentrations diffuses into the tissues causing jaundice.

Laboratory tests

The routine screening tests for liver function will be found in Chapter 1. Here those liver function tests will be discussed that may be additionally required depending on anatomy and physiology, such as those employed in the differential diagnosis of hepatocellular disease and jaundice.

As with the thyroid function tests, there are liver function tests. The best example of these are the turbidity tests, which have in the past been very important in the differential diagnosis of liver disease. However, with the current advances and the nonspecificity of these tests, they have been discarded. An order for cephalin flocculation and turbidity tests is seldom seen anymore.

NORMAL SERUM BILIRUBIN

Direct or conjugated: up to 0.3 mg/dl
Indirect or unconjugated: 0.1-1.0 mg/dl
Total: 0.1-1.2 mg/dl

NORMAL URINE UROBILINOGEN

2 hr: 0.3-1.0 Ehrlich units
24 hr: 0.05-2.5 mg/24 hr or
0.5-4.0 Ehrlich units/24 hr

NORMAL FECAL UROBILINOGEN

75-350 mg/100 gm of stool

Liver function tests in the jaundiced patient

Since bilirubin is liberated when erythrocytes are destroyed, any condition that increases erythrocyte destruction results in hemolytic jaundice. In such a case, the serum enzymes (SGOT and SGPT) are normal. There is an increase in unconjugated (indirect) bilirubin in the serum and a mild to moderate increase in urobilinogen in the urine. There is a significantly increased fecal urobilinogen, which is probably the most important single differential test in jaundice. With this, other evidence of hemolysis should be looked for, such as reticulocytosis and dropping hematocrit.

There are two rare conditions associated with an elevation of unconjugated (indirect) bilirubin from hepatic sources. They are the Crigler-Najjar syndrome and Gilbert's syndrome, in which all of the liver function tests are normal except for a slight increase in fecal urobilinogen.

Conjugated (direct) bilirubin is elevated significantly in the blood in hepatic jaundice. This condition can be caused by a virus, toxic hepatitis, acute alcoholic hepatitis, and so forth. In these cases there is extreme elevation of the liver enzymes (SGOT and SGPT), a moderate increase in alkaline phosphatase levels, and the urine urobilinogen may or may not be increased. The fecal urobilinogen is normal. The cholesterol level is somewhat diminished, particularly the esterified fraction.

A marked elevation of alkaline phosphatase, particularly in primary biliary cirrhosis is manifested in obstructive jaundice (hepatocanalicular or so-called cholestatic jaundice). Bilirubin is present in the urine and the urobilinogen level is normal, elevated, or decreased. The enzymes (SGOT and SGPT) are slightly elevated, but much less so than in acute viral or hepatocellular jaundice.

In the case of posthepatic obstruction such as a tumor of the ampulla of Vater, a carcinoma of the head of the pancreas, or a big stone in the major common bile duct, there is complete absence of fecal urobilinogen. This gives the clay color to the stools. The cholesterol is increased. The alkaline phosphatase is markedly increased. The enzyme levels (SGOT and SGPT) are mildly to moderately elevated.

Summary. In the differential diagnosis of jaundice three sets of tests are important:

1. Evidence of hepatocellular damage is reflected by the enzymes, which are elevated markedly in hepatocellular jaundice.
2. In obstructive jaundice there is extreme elevation of alkaline phosphatase, the presence of cholesterol, and the near absence of fecal urobilinogen.
3. In both hepatocellular and obstructive jaundice the most highly elevated test results are the cholesterol level and the alkaline phosphatase level. A marked elevation of direct-acting bilirubin will be present especially in obstructive jaundice.

Liver function tests not directly related to differential diagnosis of jaundice

Sulfobromophthalein excretion test (Bromsulphalein, BSP). This is a relatively simple test that should be done on a patient who is not jaundiced. A general screening test for overall liver function, it gives some indication of hepatocellular damage and cell loss and is an index to the extent of parenchymal disease. The results can also be elevated in metastatic tumors or partial obstructive situations due to tumors. The BSP dye is administered intravenously and is almost completely cleared from the blood by the normal liver.

Serum enzyme assays. *Serum alkaline phosphatase* is one of the most important determinations in the differential diagnosis of obstructive jaundice. For all practical purposes, a normal alkaline phosphatase strongly suggests liver pathology other than obstruction. Normal values are listed in Chapter 1 and Appendix A.

5-Nucleotidase is measured in conjunction with alkaline phosphatase because it is not related to bone destruction, as is alkaline phosphatase, and is not elevated in bone disease. However, it is not as specific as alkaline phosphatase in diagnosing obstructive jaundice.

NORMAL SERUM 5-NUCLEOTIDASE

0-1.6 units

The *transaminases*, serum glutamic-oxaloacetic transaminase (SGOT) and serum glutamic-pyruvic transaminase (SGPT), are liberated from destroyed cells. SGOT is found particularly in skeletal muscles, cardiac muscle, and liver while SGPT is found in liver tissue. In the absence of cardiac or other muscle injury, the elevations of SGOT and SGPT are diagnostic or hepatocellular damage in which case they are both extremely elevated.

NORMAL SERUM SGPT

1-36 U/ml

NORMAL SERUM SGOT

8-33 U/ml

Lactic dehydrogenase (LDH) is not very helpful in the diagnosis of liver disease because it is found in all organs and released into the circulation from a variety of tissue injuries. See p. 15 or Appendix A for normal values.

Serum protein. Serum protein determination is important because albumin is synthesized in the liver, and because serum globulins are produced by Kupffer cells. Therefore in typical chronic liver disease, the albumin/globulin ratio is reversed with diminution of albumin and elevation of globulin, which is a broad gamma type of elevation.

Neoplastic and inflammatory diseases of the liver produce elevation of the alpha 2 globulin fraction and sometimes biliary obstruction shows elevation in the beta globulin levels. Please see p. 12 or Appendix A for normal values.

Although this is a good screening test for overall extensive liver disease, the influence of nonhepatic factors on protein metabolism should be remembered.

Prothrombin time and vitamin K administration test. The increase of prothrombin time in liver disease may be the result of either malabsorption of the fat-soluble vitamin K or a deficiency in the formation of one of the clotting factors. The prolongation of prothrombin time would be manifested by bleeding tendencies.

The differential diagnosis of obstructive versus hepatocellular damage is made by giving an intramuscular injection of vitamin K. If the prothrombin time returns to a normal level, the implication is that the patient has obstructive problems rather than hepatocellular damage. However, if there is a continued elevation of prothrombin time, the indication is severe hepatocellular damage.

NORMAL PROTHROMBIN TIME

12-14 sec

Blood lipid and cholesterol. Blood lipid and cholesterol levels are usually elevated in obstructive jaundice and particularly in Zieve's syndrome (fatty liver), in which case there is extreme elevation of cholesterol and triglycerides. In chronic liver disease cholesterols are diminished. In both obstructive and chronic liver disease the esterified percentage of cholesterol is diminished. Please see p. 75 or Appendix A for normal values.

Blood ammonia levels. Blood ammonia levels are elevated in marked liver cirrhosis, especially following GI bleeding. This occurs because ammonia is usually metabolized to urea in the liver and is then excreted as blood urea nitrogen. However, in the presence of marked liver disease, elevated ammonia levels would be experienced. It has been suspected that some of the hepatic encephalopathy is probably a result of a high ammonia level in the cerebrospinal fluid, which injures the central nervous system. In association with elevated ammonia, blood urea nitrogen will also be diminished.

NORMAL PLASMA AMMONIA

20-150 mcg dl (diffusion)
40-80 mcg/dl (enzymatic method)
12-48 mcg/dl (resin method)

Radioisotope liver scan. This is a relatively recent scanning method in which radioactive gamma-emitting isotopes are injected intravenously and subsequently are extracted selectively by the liver. This is followed by radiation scanning of the upper abdomen, which demonstrates the patchy distribution of liver cirrhosis or a space-occupying lesion in which there is a specific area of decreased uptake of the radioactive material. Thus this test is helpful in diagnosing localizing tumors for future biopsy purposes, abscesses, and generalized nonspecific disease of the liver.

Percutaneous needle liver biopsy. Percutaneous biopsy is a safe method of establishing the pathologic and microscopic picture of the liver cell. It is most useful in the diagnosis of diffuse parenchymal disorders of the liver. It is also helpful in differentiating disseminated granulomatous focal disease from tumors.

The major indications for needle biopsy are:
1. Unexplained hepatomegaly and hepatosplenomegaly
2. Abnormal persistent liver function test
3. Suspected systemic or infiltrative disease
4. Sarcoidosis or miliary tuberculosis
5. Suspected primary or metaststic liver malignancy

Needle biopsy should not be performed if the prothrombin time is markedly elevated, if there is tense ascites, or if the patient cannot hold the breath and is uncooperative. All of these conditions increase the risk of severe bleeding.

Peritoneoscopy. This is a useful but not a routinely employed way of studying patients with liver disease. The procedure is performed by introducing the peritoneoscope into the peritoneal cavity and thus directly visualizing the gallbladder, liver, and serosal lining with a minimum of discomfort and hazard to the patient. It is additionally helpful in determining the site for the liver biopsy, which can be performed under peritoneoscopy.

SOME SPECIAL TESTS OF CURRENT INTEREST AND APPLICABILITY EMPLOYED IN GASTROENTEROLOGY
Serum gastrin level

Hypergastrinemia is one of the main characteristics of the Zollinger-Ellison syndrome, which is always accompanied by a marked increase in gastric acid secretion. A marked elevation of gastrin is present also in pernicious anemia. This probably reflects the characteristic failure of patients with this disorder to secrete gastric hydrochloric acid, which is a potent, normal inhibitor of gastrin release.

Gastrin release is slightly elevated in the fasting serum of patients with gastric ulcer disease. Also, there is a slight elevation of gastrin levels in duodenal ulcer. However, it rarely reaches the levels found in the Zollinger-Ellison syndrome.

There is significant diminution of gastric acid in gastric carcinoma. Thus, by the same mechanism of reciprocity, there will be increased gastrin secretion. In the Zollinger-Ellison syndrome, although there is high gastric acidity, which would normally suppress the gastrin secretion, there is an extremely high gastrin level, which indicates an autonomous tumor producing the excess gastrin.

NORMAL SERUM GASTRIN

40-150 pg/ml

Carcinoembryonic antigen

Initially the carcinoembryonic antigen was thought to be relatively specific for carcinoma of the GI tract, including the liver and pancreas. However, later it was found that this antigen is relatively nonspecific. In clinical practice at the present time, the role of carcinoembryonic antigen is restricted mainly to follow-up studies. If a patient with known carcinoma has an elevated carcinoembryonic antigen level preoperatively, and if this level drops postoperatively, the patient can very well be followed by this test. If there is a recurrence of elevation of the antigen, it is a good indication of recurrence of the carcinoma. However, in itself, since so many factors will cause an elevation, it is considered a nonspecific test and is not used for a definitive diagnosis of carcinoma of the GI tract.

Alpha fetoprotein ("fetal" alpha$_1$ globulin)

This is a unique protein found in the blood in carcinoma of the liver. If it is positive, if it is detected in the blood of a patient with chronic liver disease, and if it persists, it is suggestive of primary carcinoma of the liver.

Australia antigen

Australia antigen was discovered when a precipitin reaction occurred between a substance in the serum of a much-transfused hemophiliac and the serum of an Australian aborigine. The material in the Australian's serum was labeled Australia antigen. Later it was found that the hepatitis associated with long incubation periods, hepatitis B, was also associated with the finding of Australia antigen in the serum.

This test has several values. Since it is found in serum hepatitis, it differentiates between serum hepatitis and orally acquired hepatitis. However, at the present time terminology has changed to hepatitis A, which has a short incubation period and is Australia antigen negative, and hepatitis B, which has a long incubation period and is Australia antigen positive.

The clinical value of this test is that hepatitis B is more severe and of longer duration than hepatitis A, carrying with it a poorer prognosis. It is also useful in screening for Australia antigen, and thus reducing the risk of transfusion-related hepatitis.

CHAPTER 8

Diagnostic tests for endocrine disorders

ANATOMY AND PHYSIOLOGY (GENERAL)

The endocrine system is a very complex system with one common denominator. The organs of the endocrine system all produce small amounts of very active chemical substances known as hormones, which alter body metabolism. Each of the hormones is manufactured by one particular organ and is secreted into the bloodstream to exert its influence on other organs or tissues ("target tissues").

The established endocrine system, illustrated in Fig. 8-1, is comprised of the following organs: anterior and posterior pituitary, thyroid, parathyroids, adrenals, pancreatic islets of Langerhans, ovaries, testes, and placenta.

Previously, the major endocrine gland was thought to be the pituitary gland. However, the central nervous system, in particular the hypothalamus, is now considered the major endocrine organ. The hypothalamus controls the pituitary through the hypothalamic releasing factors. These releasing factors stimulate the secretion of already formed pituitary hormones. The pituitary hormones in turn stimulate various peripheral endocrine organs. The relationships of the pituitary gland and hypothalamus to the target organs are shown in Fig. 8-2. The pituitary gland is protected in the bony cavity of the sella turcica and is covered by the dura mater. The hypothalamic region is attached to the pituitary gland by a stalk, and the two act together to control the functions of the target organs. Two hypothalamic hormones have been identified: the gonadotropin-releasing factor and the thyrotropin-releasing factor, both of which cause the release of a specific pituitary hormone.

The six known hormones secreted by the anterior lobe of the pituitary gland are:
1. Growth hormone (GH), which has a general effect on growth
2. Prolactin, which controls the secretion of milk by the mammary glands
3. Thyroid-stimulating hormone (TSH), which stimulates the release and formation of thyroid hormones
4. Adrenocorticotropic hormone (ACTH), which controls the secretion of the adrenal cortex

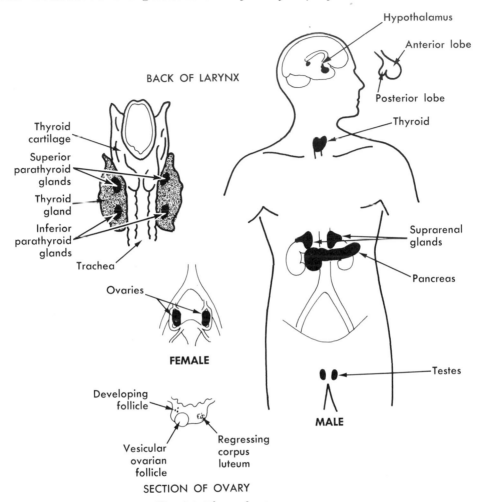

Fig. 8-1. The endocrine system.

5. Luteinizing hormone (LH), which initiates ovulation and luteinization in the ovary
6. Follicle-stimulating hormone (FSH), which stimulates estrogen secretion and the growth of the graafian follicle in women and spermatogenesis in men

The posterior pituitary hormones are vasopressin (antidiuretic hormone, ADH) and oxytocin, which are manufactured in the hypothalamus and stored in and released from the posterior pituitary gland.

The endocrine system has inherent checks and balances so that most of the endocrine function tests depend not only on excess production or underproduction of a particular hormone, but also on the reciprocal changes of one hormone production effect on others. For example, excess cortisone production from the adrenal glands suppresses ACTH by from the pituitary gland. There is then a differential diagnosis as to where the main pathology exists.

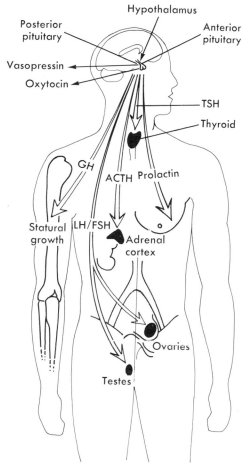

Fig. 8-2. The interrelationships between the pituitary gland, the hypothalamus, and the target organs.

THE THYROID GLAND
Anatomy and physiology

The thyroid gland (Fig. 8-3) consists of two lobes with a connecting portion (isthmus), giving the gland an H-shaped appearance. There is one lobe on each side of the trachea. This gland is unique among the endocrine glands because of its large amount of stored hormone and its slow rate of excretion.

The principal hormones secreted by the thyroid are *thyroxine* (T_4) and *triiodo-thyronine* (T_3). These hormones stimulate the oxidative reactions of most of the cells of the body, help to regulate lipid and carbohydrate metabolism, and are necessary for the normal growth and development of the organism. Most of the action of the thyroid hormone is mediated through the sympathetic nervous system. This is why beta blockers are used for hyperthyroidism.

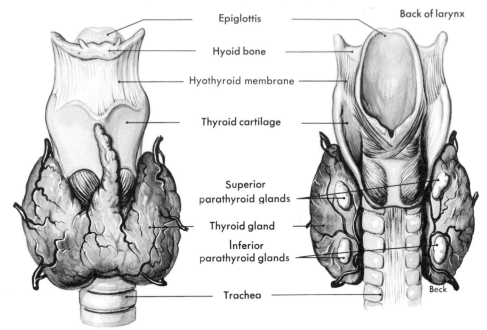

Fig. 8-3. The thyroid and parathyroid glands. (From Anthony, C. P., and Kolthoff, N. J.: Text-book of anatomy and physiology, ed. 9, St. Louis, 1975, The C. V. Mosby Co.)

The first step in the synthesis of the thyroid hormone is absorption of dietary iodide from the small intestine into the circulation. The circulating iodide that is not taken up by the thyroid gland is cleared by the kidneys through glomerular filtration. After entering the thyroid, iodide is oxidized and combines with the amino acid, tyrosine, within the protein molecule thyroglobulin, where the thyroid hormones triiodothyronine (T_3) and thyroxine (T_4) are formed.

The next step is the release of T_3 and T_4 from the thyroid gland. Under the influence of the thyroid-stimulating hormone (TSH) from the anterior pituitary gland, thyroglobulin is hydrolyzed and T_3 and T_4 are released into the circulation. Of the circulating thyroid hormones, 99.95% of the T_4 and 99.5% of the T_3 is bound to serum proteins, particularly to thyroxine-binding globulin (TBG). These hormones are inactive when bound to serum proteins. Therefore, only very small amounts of unbound thyroid hormone circulate to provide biologic activity. Although the proportion of unbound T_3 in the serum is greater than that of unbound T_4, there is more total circulating T_4. Thus, the protein-bound hormones are, therefore, more likely to reflect T_4 levels. However T_3 is four times more potent than T_4 and only one sixth less plentiful in the unbound state.

The regulation of the thyroid gland occurs through a feedback system (Fig. 8-4) consisting of three main components: (1) the thyroid gland, which secretes T_3 and T_4, (2) the anterior pituitary gland, which secretes the thyroid-stimulating hormone (TSH), and (3) the hypothalamus, which secretes thyrotropin-releasing factor (TRF).

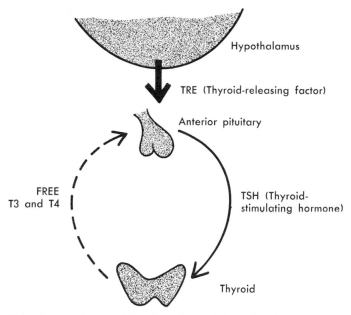

Fig. 8-4. The regulation of the thyroid gland through a feedback system.

TRF then stimulates the release of TSH and causes the synthesis of new TSH in the pituitary gland.

Normal levels of unbound T_3 and T_4 are maintained by a negative feedback effect. Increased free hormone causes decreased TSH secretion and decreased free hormone causes increased TSH secretion.

Laboratory tests for thyroid function

A multitude of new tests that are based on secretion rate, stimulation, and suppression has been developed in the past few years. The basal metabolic rate (BMR) is no longer considered *the* test for thyroid disease; in its place is a whole complex of thyroid function tests. New techniques for the identification of the thyroid hormones have been developed in the last few years, resulting in a more specific and accurate determination of the metabolically active thyroid hormone factors.

Basal metabolic rate (BMR)

In the past the most important thyroid function test was the basal metabolic rate. A low level BMR indicated hypothyroidism that was associated with hypercholesterolemia. These measurements plus the clinical picture were sufficient reason to initiate therapy.

Protein bound iodine (PBI)

With the discovery of protein bound iodine in 1950 and the introduction of radioactive iodine uptake of the thyroid gland, the BMR became obsolete. At that time there was widespread use of the PBI and the RAI uptake. However, the PBI as a thyroid function test was known to be limited, particularly because any condition that increases or decreases the proteins that carry thyroxine also falsely increases or decreases the PBI. In addition, exogenous iodine preparations interfered extensively with the test. Thus, the value of the PBI test remains limited.

Radioactive iodine (RAI)

The radioactive iodine or ^{131}I test is still used. A small tracer dose of [131]l is given intravenously and the amount that enters the gland provides an indirect measure of thyroid activity. It has, however, become less specific, particularly in detecting hypothyroid states, because of the increased use of iodinized food that suppresses the RAI uptake.

Butanol-extractable iodine (BEI)

As a slight improvement on the measurement of serum PBI, the measurement of butanol-extractable iodine was introduced during the early 1950s. This test eliminated exogenous contamination with iodine. However, it is a time-consuming and technically difficult test and does not solve the most common problem in testing thyroid function: interference from organic iodides.

Serum thyroxine (T_4) determination

The most dramatic improvement in thyroid function tests occurred between 1960 and 1966 with the development of a direct determination test of thyroxine, effectively eliminating the problem of exogenous or iodine contamination. The test is also known as the Murphy-Pattee and $T_4(D)$ (T_4 by displacement). It is a radiochemical procedure that measures the ability of serum T_4 to displace radioactive thyroxine from thyroxine-binding globulin (TBG). The development of this test was motivated by the recognition of the specificity of thyroxine-binding protein. This method is absolutely specific for thyroxine and therefore free from all iodine interference. It is, however, affected by thyroxine-binding globulin (TBG), which, if elevated, will give elevated T_4 results.

Serum triiodothyronine (T_3) determination

Soon after the introduction of the T_4 determination, a technique for the estimation of T_3 was developed. T_3 is much less stable than T_4 and occurs in very small quantities in the active form. Yet the ability to measure T_3 in the serum is clinically important when the patient has all of the symptoms of hyperthyroidism but a normal serum T_4. In such a patient, T_3 measurements may identify a T_3 thyrotoxicosis, a very rare clinical entity. There are two methods available for its measurement: (1) T_3 by displacement, which involves competitive protein binding and (2) T_3 by radioimmunoassay (T_3 [RiA]), an elaborate antigen-antibody reaction requiring special reagents that are not widely available.

Free thyroxine index

It is the free, unbound thyroxine that enters the cell, is metabolically active, and is not affected by TBG abnormalities. This is, therefore, the measurement that would be of most diagnostic value. It was found that the multiplication of the T_4 Murphy-Pattee method and the T_3 determined either by radioimmunoassay method or competitive binding displacement method correlated very well with the free thyroxine level in the serum. Thus evolved the concept of the free thyroxine index, a figure that most accurately reflects the circulating thyroid hormone, which is not affected by exogenous iodine or thyroxine-binding globulin.

Comparison of T_4, T_3, and free thyroxine

At the present time, the most useful and accurate tests for evaluating thyroid function are the T_4 determination (Murphy-Pattee) and the T_3 determination (either by displacement or radioimmunoassay method). The free thyroxine index can then be calculated. Radioactive iodine uptake is also employed in situations in which the T_3 and T_4 results are borderline or do not fit into the clinical picture.

NORMAL SERUM THYROID HORMONE

	Expressed as thyroxine	*Expressed as iodine*
T_4 (by column)	5.0-11.0 mcg/dl	3.2 7.2 mcg/dl
T_4 (by competitive binding—Murphy-Pattee)	6.0-11.8 mcg/dl	3.9-7.7 mcg/dl
Free T_4	0.9-2.3 ng/dl	0.6-1.5 ng/dl
T_3 (resin uptake)	25-35 relative % uptake	
Thyroxine-binding globulin (TBG)	10-26 mcg/dl (expressed as T_4 uptake)	

Thyroid scan

The thyroid scan is of greatest value in studying solitary thyroid nodules. Radioactive iodine is injected intravenously, after which the overall pattern of thyroid gland radioactivity can be visualized. Thus hyperactive and hypoactive areas can be localized, and the size of the gland can be determined. Hyperactive areas will indicate a hyperfunctioning nodule ("hot nodule"), and will thus differentiate between diffuse hyperplasia and toxic nodule as a cause of thyrotoxicosis. Hypoactive areas indicate a hypofunctioning nodule ("cold nodule") and thus increase the suspicion of carcinoma. The hot nodule is seldom malignant. Also, thyroid scanning provides some guidelines for therapy in hyperthyroidism when ^{131}I therapy is contemplated.

Measurement of serum thyroid-stimulating hormone

The most reliable and accurate test for primary hypothyroidism is the measurement of the thyroid-stimulating hormone, which is elevated in this condition A normal serum TSH excludes primary hypothyroidism, because an absence of thyroid hormone in the serum stimulates the pituitary gland to produce more than the normal amount of TSH.

Thyroid stimulating-hormone suppression test

This test is used to rule out hyperthyroidism. It is, however, not of value in making the diagnosis of hypothyroidism. The test is based on suppressing the thyroid-stimulating hormone by giving the patient oral T_3, the most active form of thyroid hormone. If this is followed by suppression of TSH, hyperthyroidism is ruled out.

Thyrotropin releasing hormone (TRH) stimulation test

The hypothalamus produces the thyrotropin-releasing hormone, which stimulates the release of TSH and causes the synthesis of new TSH in the pituitary gland. This test, therefore, measures diminished pituitary TSH reserve. The response to TRH stimulation is supranormal in patients with hypothyroidism of thyroid origin, whereas little or no response occurs in patients with thyrotoxicosis. This lack of response is an excellent test to confirm thyrotoxicosis. The test is also of value in the recognition and differential diagnosis of pituitary and hypothalamic hypothyroidism. In the former no response to TRH stimulation is expected.

Summary of thyroid tests

The most accurate and most commonly used tests for evaluating thyroid function at the present time are:
1. T_4 (Murphy-Pattee) method, which is also officially designated as $T_4(D)$
2. T_3 determination
3. Free thyroxine index

To further test the homeostatic controls and feedbacks, sophisticated tests employed are:
1. TSH stimulation
2. TSH suppression
3. TRH stimulation

Of historical value only is the determination of protein bound iodine (PBI), butanol-extractable iodine (BEI), and basal metabolic rate (BMR).

The thyroid scan is still the most valid test for detecting hot or cold nodules of the thyroid. For medullary carcinoma of the thyroid, increased concentration of calcitonin in the serum is diagnostic.

THE PARATHYROID GLANDS
Anatomy and physiology

There are four small parathyroid glands so closely associated with the thyroid that for some time they were often removed during thyroidectomy (Fig. 8-3). The parathyroid hormone is essential for life and is responsible for the maintenance of ionized calcium in the blood as well as for the renal excretion of calcium and phosphate.

Low serum calcium levels, by a feedback system, trigger an increase in the production of the parathyroid hormone, which acts on the bone, kidney, and intestine to increase serum calcium. Osteoclasts, in response to the parathyroid hormone, release bone salts into the extracellular fluid, thereby raising both calcium and phosphate levels in the plasma. The renal tubular cells, in response to the parathyroid hormone, increase reabsorption of calcium and decrease reabsorption of phosphate from the glomerular filtrate.

Calcitonin, a potent hypocalcemic hormone, has effects opposing those of the parathyroid hormone because it increases renal calcium clearance.

Vitamin D also plays an important role in calcium homeostasis by increasing the efficiency of intestinal calcium absorption.

Evaluation of parathyroid function was discussed in Unit I in the section on calcium and phosphate. Hypercalcemia is still essential for the diagnosis of hyperparathyroidism. However, additional tests that have also been advocated will be discussed.

Laboratory tests

Tests for hyperparathyroidism in addition to serum calcium determination

Phosphate clearance. This is not a very accurate test and has many variables. Excessive parathyroid hormone accompanied by an increase in phosphate excretion provides the physiologic basis for the test.

Phosphate reabsorption test. The parathyroid hormone prevents renal tubular reabsorption of phosphorus. The phosphate reabsorption test is accomplished by comparing the creatinine clearance with the phosphate clearance. This comparison gives the amount of phosphate reabsorbed by the tubules per minute, and is therefore some indication of the level of parathyroid hormone in the serum.

Additional tests. Phosphate loading tests and calcium infusion tests have been advocated in the past but have not been too reliable. Also attempts have been made at parathyroid scanning and arteriography, though they are not clinically applicable at the present time. In certain cases therapeutic responses to glucocorticosteroids have been employed. This procedure is helpful in the differential diagnosis since the glucocorticosteroids generally do not affect the calcium levels in hyperparathyroidism but do suppress the majority of hypercalcemias of other etiologies.

It is also known that thiazide diuretics given to patients with hyperparathyroidism increase the serum calcium level.

Recently made available is the immunoassay method of measuring the parathyroid hormone level in the blood. Soon this test will probably be the most important diagnostic test for parathyroid function.

Tests for hypoparathyroidism

Hypoparathyroidism is uncommon. Tests recently advocated to diagnose hypoparathyroidism include parathyroid hormone (parathormone) assay, which is not readily available, and urinary levels of cyclic AMP following treatment with parathormone. At the present time these tests are too new for use in routine clinical practice.

Test for metastatic carcinoma to bone

Bone scanning. Bone scanning is used to detect metastatic carcinoma to bone. A radioactive isotope of elements that are involved in bone metabolism is used to detect the foci of metastatic tumors in advance of detection by x-ray films.

THE ADRENAL GLANDS
Anatomy and physiology

A right and a left adrenal gland overlap the upper ends of the kidneys. These glands are composed of two distinct parts, the medullary or inner portion and the cortical or outer portion (Fig. 8-5). The adrenal medulla secretes the catecholamines, epinephrine and norepinephrine. The adrenal cortex secretes the steroid hormones.

The adrenocortical hormones

The steroid hormones of the adrenal cortex and their physiologic effects (Fig. 8-6) are:
1. The glucocorticoids, *cortisol* and corticosterone, which affect metabolism of proteins, carbohydrates and lipids
2. The mineralocorticoid, *aldosterone*, which predominantly affects sodium and potassium excretion
3. The sex steroids, androgens or estrogens, which primarily affect secondary sex characteristics

Terminology

An understanding of a portion of the biochemistry and physiology of steroids is helpful.

The carbon atoms on the basic steroid nucleus are numbered in sequence from 1 to 17. The steroids derived from this basic nucleus are of two structural types, the C-19 steroids and the C-21 steroids.

The C-19 steroids have predominantly androgenic activity and carry methyl groups at positions C-18 and C-10. If there is also a ketone group at the C-17 position, they are called *17-ketosteroids.*

The C-21 steroids have predominantly either glucocorticoid or mineralocorticoid properties and have 2-carbon side chains (C-20 and C-21) attached at position 17 of the molecule. There are also methyl groups at C-18 and C-19. The C-21 steroids that also possess a hydroxyl group at position 17 of the steroid nucleus are called *17-hydroxycorticosteroids (or 17-hydroxycorticoids).*

Adrenocorticotrophic hormone (ACTH)

The role of the anterior pituitary gland in adrenal cortical secretion is displayed in Fig. 8-7. Adrenocorticotrophic hormone is stored in and released from the anterior pituitary gland. The release of stored ACTH is governed by a corticotropin-releasing factor (CRF) in the hypothalamus, which is in turn governed by plasma cortisol levels, stress, and the sleep-wake cycle. The plasma ACTH level roughly follows a diurnal pattern, being highest just prior to waking and lowest just prior to retiring. In certain types of stress (emotional trauma, surgery, pyrogens) the ACTH levels rise. However, the circulating cortisol is the principal regulator of ACTH and CRF release. This is a negative feedback mechanism (Fig. 8-6) that, when plasma cortisol is low, causes a release of CRF. When plasma cortisol is high there is a decrease in the release of CRF.

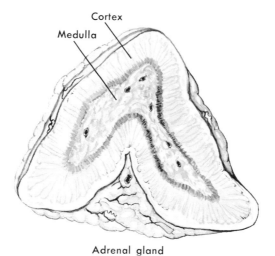

Fig. 8-5. The adrenal gland. (From Schottelius, B. A., and Schottelius, D. D.: Textbook of physiology, ed. 17, St. Louis, 1973, The C. V. Mosby Co.)

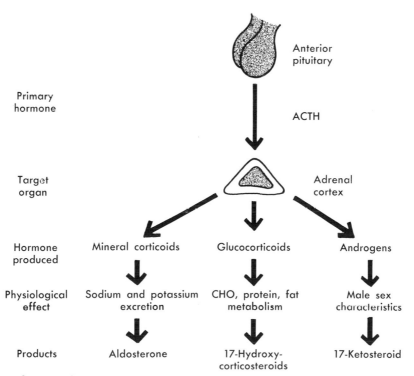

Fig. 8-6. The steroid hormones of the adrenal cortex, their physiological effects and products.

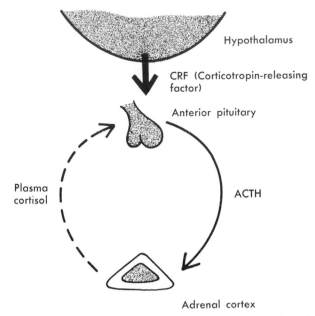

Fig. 8-7. The role of the hypothalamus and anterior pituitary gland in adrenal cortical secretion.

Aldosterone

Aldosterone, a mineralocorticoid secreted by the adrenal cortex, is the chief electrolyte-regulating hormone of the adrenal gland. The kidneys require aldosterone for the normal reabsorption of sodium, which leads to a secondary loss of potassium. Normally an increase in serum sodium triggers a decrease in the rate of aldosterone secretion, causing the kidney to lose large quantities of sodium until the serum sodium is back to normal. Conversely, if the serum sodium falls below normal or if serum potassium rises, the rate of aldosterone secretion increases so that sodium is retained and potassium lost.

Aldosterone secretion is also under the control of the hormone renin, which is secreted by the kidney cells in hypovolemic or hyponatremic states. The renin-angiotensin-aldosterone system is described on p. 110.

Laboratory tests for adrenocortical function

Adrenal function tests are divided into two major categories, (1) absolute determination of individual hormone values in both the serum and the urine, and (2) tests that reflect the interdependency of one hormone on another and feedback mechanisms.

Until a few years ago the steroid determinations were performed only on highly selected patients in major medical centers. However, with present technology, these tests are no longer confined only to the major medical centers.

Absolute determination of individual adrenal hormone values

Plasma cortisol levels. Cortisol, the most potent glucocorticoid, is also the most abundant of the major circulating adrenocorticosteroids.

Plasma cortisol levels are obtained in the morning and also in the evening, preferably at 8 A.M. and 8 P.M. In the healthy person the secretion rate is higher in the early morning hours and lower in the evening hours. This diurnal variation is interrupted if there is any disturbance of the hypothalamo-pituitary axis or if there is an autonomous lesion in the adrenals producing the excess cortisol levels. Extreme elevation of the plasma cortisol level without diurnal variation is very suggestive of autonomous carcinoma.

NORMAL PLASMA CORTISOL

8 A.M.-10 A.M.: 5-25 mcg/dl
4 P.M.- 6 P.M.: 2-18 mcg/dl

24 hour urine steroids. The next best test for evaluating adrenal function is the 24-hour collection of urine for hydroxycorticosteroids and ketosteroids. The principal determinations with normal values appear below.

17-hydroxycorticosteroids (17-hydroxycorticoids). These steroids are measured in a 24-hour urine specimen as Porter-Silber chromogens. (The Porter-Silber reaction is a sensitive index of adrenocortical function.) The 17-hydroxycorticoids include the C-17, C-20, and C-21 hydroxysteroids, that is those steroids with hydroxyl groups on C-17 (carbon number 17), a ketone group on C-20, and C-21.

Elevated hydroxycorticoisteroids in the urine usually indicate either primary or secondary hyperadrenalism, and elevated ketogenic steroids have more or less the same implication.

NORMAL 17-HYDROXYCORTICOSTEROIDS (24 HOUR URINE)

Male: 5.5-14.5 mg/24 hr
Female: 4.9-12.9 mg/24 hr
Lower in children
After 25 USP units ACTH, I.M.: a two-fold to fourfold increase

17-ketosteroids. The urine 17-ketosteroids are those C-19 steroids that also contain a ketone group at C-17 (carbon number 17) of the steroid nucleus. They are determined by the Zimmerman reaction.

Extreme elevation of the 17-ketosteroids suggests an autonomous tumor that is secreting mainly androgenic steroids. Ketosteroids are also elevated in virilizing syndromes, particularly in the adrenogenital syndrome. In such a situation, also an elevation of urinary pregnanetriol and pregnanediol.

NORMAL 17-KETOSTEROIDS (24 HOUR URINE)

Male: 8-15 mg/24 hr
Female: 6-11.5 mg/24 hr
Children (12-15 yr): 5-12 mg/24 hr
(<12 yr): <5 mg/24 hr
After 25 USP units ACTH, I.M.: 50%-100% increase

Ketogenic steroids. This term refers to the C-21 hydroxycorticoids that can be oxidized to 17-ketosteroids in vitro and thus can be measured by the Zimmerman reaction.

NORMAL 24 HOUR URINE KETOGENIC STEROIDS

5-23 mg/24 hr

Aldosterone levels. Usually, aldosterone levels are ordered in hypertensive patients. At the present time hypertensive patients are being classified as high-aldosterone, high-renin producers or as high-aldosterone producers without high-renin production. The latter group is considered to have relatively benign hypertension, whereas the high-renin, high-aldosterone producers are thought to be vulnerable to the vascular catastrophies associated with hypertension and vascular disease. Aldosterone determination is, therefore, becoming very important. It should be performed under controlled situations in which the sodium and potassium intakes, as well as the supine and standing states, are closely monitored, because a potent stimulus to the release of renin is a low sodium diet for four to five days followed by a four-hour period in the upright posture.

NORMAL PLASMA ALDOSTERONE

0.015 mcg/100 ml

NORMAL 24 HOUR URINE ALDOSTERONE

2-26 mcg/24 hr

Elevated aldosterone levels. Elevated aldosterone levels can be found in primary aldosteronism resulting from aldosterone-producing adenomas or hyperfunction of the aldosterone-producing cells of the adrenals.

Secondary aldosteronism, in which the aldosterone is usually increased secondary to renin production, may also be a cause of elevated aldosterone levels.

Elevated aldosterone may also be a result of increased ACTH production. However, this mechanism does not seem to be the major factor in the production of aldosterone.

At the present time tests to determine aldosterone levels are not performed routinely in hypertensive patients. However, it seems reasonable that they will be performed routinely as a criterion in the selection of appropriate treatment, since renin suppression may be the treatment of choice in certain types of hypertension, whereas aldosterone suppression would be the treatment in other types.

Plasma ACTH levels. Adrenocorticotrophic hormone (ACTH), also known as the adrenocortical-stimulating hormone, governs the secretion of glucocorticoids and the sympathetic response to stress from the adrenal glands.

ACTH levels are elevated when there is primary adrenal deficiency, particularly of the hydrocorticosteroid levels, causing the reciprocal elevation of plasma ACTH.

Extremely high levels of ACTH are found in ectopic ACTH-producing tumors or in pituitary adenomas in which there is increased secretion of ACTH.

NORMAL PLASMA ACTH AT 8 A.M.

< 150 pg/ml

Feedback mechanisms and tests that reflect interdependency of hormones

These tests measure, by means of stimulation and suppression, the integrity of the functions of the hypothalamus and the pituitary and adrenal glands.

ACTH stimulation test. The ACTH stimulation test demonstrates the ability of the adrenal glands to produce steroids. Forty units of ACTH is infused within eight hours. If the patient responds with an increase in plasma cortisol levels, the disease is secondary and not primary adrenal related. This test is not of much clinical help.

Aldosterone stimulation test. One of the best stimulators of aldosterone secretion is the lowering of serum sodium level. This can be accomplished with a potent diuretic such as furosemide (Lasix), which will significantly stimulate aldosterone production, or with a low sodium diet.

Glucocorticoid suppression tests. Dexamethasone (Decadron) is a synthetic steroid with actions similar to, but much more potent than, cortisone. Therefore, very small doses suppress pituitary ACTH production, which is reflected in the urine by decreased corticosteroids.

The dexamethasone suppression test is probably the most widely used, practical, and informative procedure available to evaluate pituitary ACTH production. At the present time the test is done overnight. Intravenous dexamethasone is given and if the 17-hydroxycorticoids are not suppressed to below 50% of the control value, a tumor is usually present.

Aldosterone suppression (desoxycorticosterone [Doca] test). The administration of desoxycorticosterone (Doca) along with large amounts of salt will suppress aldosterone production. If the patient has primary aldosteronism there is little or no suppression, but a patient with essential hypertension has a suppression of greater than 50%, which is the normal suppression.

The Doca is administered intramuscularly, 10 mg every twelve hours for three days. Urinary aldosterone measurements of 24 hour specimens collected before Doca administration and after the final injection on the third day are performed.

Adrenal medullary tests

The adrenal medulla is a part of the sympathetic nervous system. It differs from other ganglia of the sympathetic nervous system because it secretes more epinephrine (adrenaline) than norepinephrine, and it secretes its hormones directly into the bloodstream, classifying it as an endocrine organ.

The adrenal medullary function is not routinely tested except when there is a clinical picture of hypertension or pheochromocytoma, a tumor of the adrenal medulla. Abnormally large amounts of catecholamines are released into the circulation in pheochromocytoma. A small percentage of these catecholamines is excreted unchanged in the urine. Some of the adrenal medullary hormones appear in the urine as metanephrine, and the major portion of the hormones will be excreted as vanillylmandelic acid (VMA). Therefore, a complete workup of a patient with possible pheochromocytoma should include a 24 hour urine collection with determinations of VMA, catecholamines, and metanephrine, any one of which might be elevated in a given case of pheochromocytoma.

THE PITUITARY GLAND
Anatomy and physiology

The pituitary gland has three lobes: anterior, intermediate, and posterior. This endocrine organ secretes at least ten hormones, almost all of which exert their effect on target organs (Fig. 8-2).

Laboratory tests for pituitary function

Most of the tests performed for pituitary function have already been described under the different target organs, the thyroid and the adrenals. An adenoma of the pituitary gland initially increases secretion by the target organ. For example, there may be an increase of thyroxine and of hydroxysteroids or ketosteroids initially due to stimulation of the thyroid and adrenal glands. Later on, as more pituitary tissue is destroyed, there is diminution of the pituitary secretions and secondary failure of the target organs.

Growth hormone measurement

The growth hormone (GH) is elevated in gigantism in children and in acromegaly in adults. This is usually the result of eosinophilic adenomas of the pituitary. Measurements of the GH are taken during the course of a glucose tolerance test, since it is important to demonstrate a lack of suppressibility of elevated GH levels with glucose administration.

Metyrapone (Metopirone) administration is a measure of pituitary responsiveness, being a selective inhibitor of one of the steps in the biosynthesis of cortisol. In the final hydroxylation reaction that forms cortisol, a blocking and a secretion of compound S instead of cortisol is present. The diminished values of cortisol stimulate the pituitary to produce ACTH in a negative feedback mechanism. In the normal individual, the administration of metyrapone should cause more ACTH production from the pituitary and result in an increase in urinary hydroxysteroids and ketosteroids.

X-ray films of the skull

It is usually advisable to take an x-ray film of the skull to evaluate the sella turcica, a depression in the sphenoid bone of the skull where the pituitary gland rests, for erosion or enlargement.

A spinal fluid examination and a measurement of the visual fields should also be performed.

Vasopressin injection

In diseases of the posterior lobe of the pituitary gland a vasopressin (antidiuretic hormone ADH) deficiency is present, manifested by excessive urine output that may amount to up to twelve to fifteen liters per day. The patient will respond to a vasopressin injection with a decrease in urine output, thus documenting the deficiency and the normal responsiveness of the renal tubules to the hormone.

Recall that ADH is secreted by the hypothalamus and posterior pituitary gland and promotes increased water reabsorption from the distal tubules and collecting ducts.

URINE AND SERUM OSMOLALITY

These tests have already been described on p. 112 of Chapter 6. Serum and urine osmolality are measured when inappropriate ADH secretion syndrome is suspected.

Normally, hyperosmolar serum stimulates the osmoreceptors and the posterior pituitary produces ADH in an attempt to dilute the blood. The individual is also thirsty, a physiologic sign of hyperosmolar blood. Conversely, when there is hypo-osmolarity ADH is not secreted and the individual excretes a diluted urine. In the so-called inappropriate ADH secretion syndrome there is hypoosmolarity of the blood in association with a relative hyperosmolarity of the urine, indicating a malfunction of the normal osmolar response of the osmoreceptors, an excess of exogenous vaso-pressin, or a production of a vasopressin-like hormone that is not under the regular control of serum osmolarity.

The inappropriate secretion of ADH has been described in multiple etiologic disease entities such as bronchogenic carcinoma or other types of cancer, in congestive heart failure and inflammatory pulmonary lesions, in some metabolic diseases such as porphyria, and in some patients with excessive diuretic use.

The diagnosis is made by simultaneous measurement of the urine and serum osmolality. The serum osmolality will be much lower than the urine osmolality, indicating the inappropriate excretion of a concentrated urine in the presence of a dilute serum.

THE HYPOGLYCEMIAS

Blood sugar determination and its importance have been discussed in the first section of the book. However, at that time the hypoglycemias were not discussed.

Clinically the following four types of hypoglycemia are most frequently en-countered.

Reactive hypoglycemia

This is the most common type of hypoglycemia and is usually seen in diabetic and some prediabetic patients. Reactive hypoglycemia is thought to be the result of inappropriate release of insulin when the blood sugar is low. It occurs because of a lag in insulin release when the blood sugar is high, causing a delayed release after the blood sugar has already started to lower.

Hypoglycemia caused by insulin-producing tumors

Insulinomas from the pancreas cause hypoglycemia. Occasionally noninsulin secreting tumors cause hypoglycemia, particularly large retroperitoneal sarcomas.

Iatrogenic hypoglycemia

Both insulin injections and long-acting oral hypoglycemics cause this type of hypoglycemia.

Alcoholic hypoglycemia

Alcoholic hypoglycemia is common in chronic alcoholics who drink for a few days without eating.

CHAPTER 9

Diagnostic tests for hematologic disorders

The anatomy and physiology of blood formation is discussed in Chapter 2.

LABORATORY TESTS
The bone marrow

The bone marrow, which produces millions of blood cells daily (hemopoiesis), is the major site of the formation of blood. In the adult the red bone marrow is found in only a few locations, mainly in the membranous bones, such as the vertebrae, the sternum, and the ribs. The most accessible region for bone marrow examination is the sternum by means of sternal puncture or the iliac crest. Since the bone marrow is the center of hemopoiesis, the system that actually produces the blood can be examined when a disorder in this production is suspected.

A bone marrow examination is diagnostic in the following diseases.

Leukemias

The examination is helpful especially if there is a differential diagnostic problem with the peripheral smear, such as leukemia versus leukemoid reaction, or in aleukemic leukemia in which the peripheral smear is not diagnostic of leukemia. In the bone marrow examination the ratio between myeloid cells and erythroid cells is decidedly increased in leukemia with an increase of early immature forms.

Iron deficiency anemia

In the early stages of iron deficiency anemia a bone marrow examination reveals normoblastic hyperplasia, but the severe iron deficiency later restricts erythropoiesis (the formation of red blood cells) to the basal level. The normoblasts are small with frayed edges. Smears stained for iron reveal storage iron to be absent.

Megaloblastosis

Although at the present time the levels of vitamin B_{12} and folic acid in the blood are being relied on increasingly for the diagnosis of macrocytic anemia, a bone marrow aspiration reveals megaloblasts in both vitamin B_{12} and folic acid deficiencies. This is diagnostic since the deficiency is responsible for the megaloblastosis.

Multiple myeloma

The bone marrow aspiration can be diagnostic in this condition, if sheaths of plasma cells occupying most of the marrow elements are seen. The plasma cells may vary from less than 1% to over 90% of marrow, depending upon the degree of involvement in the site of marrow aspirated.

Hemolytic anemias

The bone marrow is important in documenting hemolysis as a possible cause of anemia, although the different causes of hemolytic anemias are not differentiated.

Hypoplastic or aplastic anemias

The diagnosis of these anemias can only be made through a bone marrow examination, which reveals hypocellularity.

Evaluation of bleeding disorders

Usually bleeding results from either failure to clot normally or failure to prevent excessive clotting due to consumption of clotting factors. An example of the first condition is excess heparin intake or some clotting factor deficiency. An example of the second condition is disseminated intravascular coagulopathy.

Theory of blood coagulation

The theory of blood coagulation should be known in order to understand the various laboratory tests designed to demonstrate defects in the coagulation mechanism.

The process of blood coagulation is one of the most complicated in the body. At least thirty five compounds take part in the formation of a firm clot, which is made up of an insoluble network of fibrous material called *fibrin*. The clotting process is divided into four stages, which are described below and illustrated in Table 9-1 along with the corresponding laboratory tests that reveal disorders in each stage. The various blood factors involved are also included in Table 9-1 (Roman numbers).

Stage I: Release of platelet factors. When blood comes in contact with a rough area on the blood vessel endothelium, such as that caused by a cut in the vessel or very commonly a patch of cholesterol-lipid substance, clumps of platelets begin to attach to the rough area within a matter of seconds. The platelet membranes then rupture and a substance is released that initiates the clotting mechanism.

Stage II: Thromboplastin generation. The platelet factors, in union with calcium ions and other coagulation factors present in normal blood, form a substance called thromboplastin.

Stage III: Conversion of prothrombin to thrombin. Thromboplastin then catalyzes the conversion of prothrombin, a circulating inactive protein, to thrombin. Calcium

Table 9-1. Theory of blood coagulation and corresponding tests

Blood coagulation	Corresponding tests and excreted results

Stage I *Platelets*
        Contact factor
	Platelet count (low)
	Clot retraction (deficient)
	Tourniquet test (positive)
	Prothrombin consumption time
	    (abnormal)

Stage II *Platelet factor* $\xrightarrow{\text{Ca}^{++}}$ Thromboplastin
        Thromboplastin   VIII
                         IX
        generation   X
        factors   XI
                         XII
	Prothrombin time (normal)
	Partial thromboplastin time
	    (abnormal)
	Prothrombin consumption time
	    (abnormal)

Stage III *Prothrombin* $\xrightarrow{\text{Ca}^{++}}$ Thrombin
        Accelerator   V
        factors   VII
                       X
	Prothrombin time (abnormal)
	Partial thromboplastin time
	    (normal)

Stage IV *Fibrinogen* $\xrightarrow{\text{XIII}}$ Fibrin	Venous clotting time (abnormal) Plasma fibrinogen (abnormal) Protamine sulfate test (abnormal) Clot lysis (abnormal)

ions are also necessary for this conversion, along with other substances known as accelerator factors. Vitamin K is necessary for the synthesis of prothrombin, which takes place in the liver.

Stage IV: Formation of fibrin. Thrombin then catalyzes the conversion of fibrinogen, another circulating inactive protein, to fibrin, the final mesh that forms the clot.

Tests in hemorrhagic disorders

Stage I. A defect in the clotting mechanism at the platelet hemolysis stage may be confirmed by the following tests.

Platelet count. Because Stage I depends on platelet clumping and hemolysis with the release of the platelet factor, a decrease in platelets affects the clotting mechanism at its initiation.

Clot retraction. Normally, after about an hour the blood clot shrinks and becomes much firmer. Platelets play a major part in the mechanism of clot retraction; therefore, a deficiency in this mechanism indicates a platelet problem (thrombocytopenia).

Tourniquet test. This test demonstrates capillary fragility caused by intrinsic defects in the capillary walls or some types of thrombocytopenia. A blood pressure cuff is inflated to maintain pressure halfway between systolic and diastolic for five minutes. A 1½ inch circle is drawn below the antecubital fossa and observed for petechiae. Normal subjects may form up to five petechiae.

Prothrombin consumption time (PCT). This test measures prothrombin utilization and is, therefore, very sensitive to defects in Stages I and II. In these two stages, a decrease in the utilization of prothrombin causes a greater amount to be left in the serum, thus shortening the serum prothrombin time.

Stage II. Defects at this stage of the clotting mechanism may be indicated by the following tests.

Prothrombin time (PT time). A calcium-binding anticoagulant is added to the patient's serum in this test. The time between the addition of the calcium and the appearance of a fibrin clot is the prothrombin time. The prothrombin time primarily shows defects in Stage III and is therefore normal when the defect is at Stage II.

Partial thromboplastin time (PTT). This test is very sensitive to defects in Stage II. It is known that although hemophiliac plasma clots normally in the presence of a potent tissue thromboplastin, it does not do so in the presence of certain incomplete or partial thromboplastins because the plasma defect of hemophilia cannot be compensated for. This test depends on a fibrin clot formation, as does the prothrombin time.

Stage III. Defects of sufficient severity at this stage of the clotting mechanism will be manifest by an abnormal prothrombin time. The partial thromboplastin time is normal unless the defect is severe. These tests are described above.

Stage IV. A defect at this stage results in an abnormal prothrombin time as well as abnormalities in the following tests.

Venous clotting time (VCT). This procedure, initially described by Lee and White in 1913, is based on the principle that whole blood, when exposed to a foreign surface, forms a solid clot. The time required for the solid clot to form is the clotting time.

Plasma fibrinogen. Normally, fibrinogen is converted to fibrin, and the clot separates from the plasma. The fibrinogen is then measured indirectly.

Clot lysis test. This test is a measure of circulating fibrinolysins, which if present in sufficient quantities can dissolve the blood clot.

Protamine sulfate test. Normally, thrombin catalyzes the conversion of fibrinogen to fibrin, which then forms the scaffolding of the blood clot. Fibrinolysins may attack either fibrinogen or fibrin to prevent the formation of the fibrin scaffolding. This test depends on the presence of the fibrin before clots are formed. Protamine sulfate acts on the fibrin and allows it to clot even in the presence of secondary fibrinolysins. However, if the fibrinolysins are primary, a protamine sulfate reaction is not elicited because there is no fibrin on which the compound may act.

Summary

If the patient has platelet count abnormalities, defective clot retraction, a positive tourniquet test, and abnormal prothrombin consumption test, the defect is most likely at Stage I.

If the patient has a normal prothrombin time and abnormal partial thromboplastin and prothrombin consumption times, the defect is at Stage II.

If the patient has an abnormal prothrombin time and normal partial thromboplastin time, the defect is at Stage III.

An abnormal venous clotting time, plasma fibrinogen level, clot lysis test, and protamine sulfate test indicate a defect at the Stage IV.

After these tests, individual factor assays must be performed to define which particular factor is involved in the defect. These assays are rarely indicated and performed only in major centers.

Blood typing and cross-matching

Before a blood transfusion is given, the blood group of the recipient and of the donor must be determined to ensure the similarity of the antigenic and immune properties of the blood of the two individuals. If the necessary precautions are not taken, red blood cell agglutination (clumping) and hemolysis (release of hemoglobin) may result. This is called a transfusion reaction and can lead to the death of the patient.

In an emergency in which there is not time to actually determine the type of antigens on the red blood cell membranes (blood type) of the donor and recipient, the bloods can be cross-matched. This procedure determines if agglutination will occur and requires mixing the cells of the donor with the defibrinated serum of the recipient. The reverse procedure is then performed: the cells of the recipient are cross-matched against the serum of the donor. The antigen is contained on the red blood cells and the antibody is contained in the serum.

Blood groups (types)

An antigen is any substance that causes formation of antibodies. The surface of the red blood cells has antigens that determine the blood type of the individual. Normally, people do not form antibodies against the antigens of their own red cells, but if a person receives a transfusion with blood containing different antigens, antibodies will be formed against all of the foreign antigens. Among the antigens, two groups, the ABO and Rh groups, are highly antigenic and can cause transfusion reactions if they are transfused into persons with incompatible blood types.

ABO blood groups. Individuals may have either A antigens, B antigens, both, or neither on their red cells. In the latter case, the blood type is usually type O.

If an individual *does not* have type A red blood cells, antibodies known as "anti-A" agglutinins will be present in the serum. If this person is transfused with type A blood, these agglutinins will agglutinate the type A red blood cells of the donor. The same is true if an individual *does not* have type B red blood cells. The serum will contain antibodies known as "anti-B" agglutinins, which will agglutinate type B red blood cells. If the individual has both A and B (AB group) antigens on the red cells, no agglutinins (antibodies) are present and the individual can receive any type of blood ("universal recipient"). If the individual is type O, with neither A nor B antigens on the red cells, the serum will contain both anti-A and anti-B agglutinins. Both A and B blood types will be agglutinated if given to the type O individual. However, since the red cells of the type O individual cannot be agglutinated by the serum of any other blood group, these persons are called universal donors.

Rh groups. Most individuals possess an antigen on their red cells called the Rh factor. These persons are said to be Rh positive, whereas those persons who do not possess the factor are said to be Rh negative. Antibodies (agglutinins) to the Rh factor do not occur spontaneously as in the ABO group. If an Rh negative individual is transfused with Rh positive blood, anti-Rh agglutinins develop slowly against the Rh positive blood. This causes no ill effects unless the person is subsequently again transfused with Rh positive blood. Then the anti-Rh agglutinins that formed in the serum as a result of the first transfusion will agglutinate the cells of the second Rh positive transfusion. Of course, Rh negative blood does no harm to an Rh positive person.

If an Rh negative mother is carrying an Rh positive fetus, the antigen from the blood cells of the fetus causes antibody production in the serum of the mother. The firstborn child usually shows no ill effects, but with subsequent pregnancies the antibodies in the mother's serum have increased and are sufficient to cause agglutination and hemolysis of the red cells of the fetus.

Hemoglobin electrophoresis

There may be two or three different types of hemoglobin in the red blood cells of an individual. The amino acid composition of the globin portion of the hemoglobin molecule is responsible for this difference. The process of filter paper electrophoresis determines the differences in the hemoglobins and identifies the abnormal hemoglobins.

In the normal adult red blood cells, hemoglobin A_1, A_2, and F are present, with only a trace of the latter two.

The most common hemoglobin abnormalities are hemoglobin S, which causes sickle cell disease if homozygous and sickle cell trait if heterozygous; and hemoglobin C disease, which may cause mild hemolytic anemia.

Coombs (antiglobulin) test

In the Coombs test antiglobulin serum is used to detect immunoglobulins (Ig) on the surface of the red cells. The antiglobulin serum is secured from a rabbit that has been injected with human globulin, and is known as Coombs serum.

In the direct Coombs test, the patient's washed red cells are mixed with Coombs serum. The mixture is then examined for agglutination. If the human red cells are coated with immunoglobulins, agglutination will occur. The test is called direct because only one step is needed—adding the Coombs serum directly to the washed cells. A positive direct Coombs test is found in hemolytic disease of the newborn, hemolytic transfusion reactions, and in idiopathic acquired hemolytic anemias.

The indirect Coombs test requires two steps. The first step may be done in one of two ways:

1. Red cells of known antigenic makeup are exposed to serum containing unknown antibodies. The second stage detects whether or not the antibody combines with the red cells. Agglutination at the second stage proves that a circulating antibody to one or more antigens on the red cells is present. The antibody may then be more specifically identified since the red cell antigens are known.
2. Red cells of unknown antigenic makeup are exposed to serum containing known

antibodies. The second stage detects whether or not the antibody combines with the red cells, thus identifying the antigen on the red cells.

In the second stage of the indirect Coombs test, Coombs serum is added to the red cells, which have been washed to remove unattached antibodies. The Coombs serum then causes agglutination if a specific antibody has coated the red cells.

The indirect Coombs test is used to detect IgG antibodies (anti-Rh_0 (D)); demonstrate autoantibodies in the serum of patients with autoimmune hemolytic anemia; demonstrate other antigen-antibody reactions involving white cells, platelets, and tissue cells; and demonstrate hypogammaglobulinemia and agammaglobulinemia.

Erythrocyte enzyme assays

At least fourteen forms of hemolytic anemia are associated with a deficiency of erythrocyte enzymes. Although quantitative assays are necessary for the identification of most of these anemias. simple screening tests are available for two of the more common forms of hemolytic anemia: glucose-6-phosphate dehydrogenase deficiency (Favism, G-6-PD) and pyruvate kinase deficiency. The screening test involves the use of long-wave ultraviolet light with which the erythrocytes are activated. Most oxidative compounds will precipitate a hemolytic crisis when these enzymes are deficient.

Osmotic fragility test

The osmotic fragility test is based on the principle that spherocytes will hemolyze in hypertonic solutions. It is positive in hereditary spherocytosis and usually negative in other hemolytic anemias.

Autohemolysis

Autohemolysis, useful when erythrocyte enzyme assays are not available, helps to differentiate between hereditary spherocytosis and congenital nonspherocytic hemolytic anemias caused by enzyme deficiency. The test is performed by measuring the amount of spontaneous hemolysis in sterile defibrinated blood that has been incubated for twenty four to forty eight hours at 37° C.

In hereditary spherocytosis the addition of ATP (adenosine triphosphate) and glucose diminishes hemolysis significantly, whereas in congenital nonspherocytic hemolytic anemias only partial reduction of hemolysis may occur.

LABORATORY TESTS IN THE CLINICAL SETTING
The hemolytic anemias

The term hemolysis refers to the destruction of red blood cells with the release of the hemoglobin into the surrounding medium. In the hemolytic anemias the life span of the red blood cells is shortened as a result of the greatly accelerated destruction of the mature red blood cells.

Diagnostic laboratory tests

Hemolysis can be documented with the appearance of bilirubinemia, reticulo-cytosis, urobilinogenemia, or urobilinogenuria.

Differential diagnosis

Hemolytic disorders may be caused by a defect in the red blood cells, which may be either congenital or acquired (vitamin B_{12} or folic acid deficiency), by factors extraneous to the red blood cells, such as transfusion incompatibility, chemical agents, and the like. The following list contains the more commonly encountered hemolytic anemias along with the laboratory tests most helpful in the differential diagnosis.

Hemolytic anemias caused by defective erythrocytes*

A. Congenital
1. Membrane defects, such as occur in hereditary spherocytosis (spherocytosis on the peripheral smear and an increase of osmotic fragility and autohemolysis)
2. Hereditary deficiencies in the Embden-Meyerhof pathway (anaerobic gly-colysis), such as occur in pyruvate kinase deficiency (low levels of erythrocyte PK shown by specific assays of the red blood cell glycolytic enzymes)
3. Abnormalities of the phosphoglucokinase oxidative pathway, such as glucose-6-phosphate dehydrogenase (G-6-PD) deficiency; more than one hundred varieties have been described; hemolysis is precipitated sometimes by the ingestion of various drugs; (erythrocyte enzyme assays)
4. Qualitative abnormalities in globin peptides—hemoglobinopathies such as hemoglobin C disease and sickle cell disease (hemoglobin electrophoresis)
5. Quantitative abnormality in globin peptide synthesis—thalassemias (hemo-globin electrophoresis shows an increase of hemoglobin F in thalassemia major, a decrease of normal hemoglobin A_1 and a relative increase of hemo-globin A_2 in thalassemia minor)

B. Acquired
1. Vitamin B_{12} deficiency (serum B_{12} levels, Schilling test)
2. Folic acid deficiency (folic acid levels)
3. Paroxysmal nocturnal hemoglobinuria (plasma hemoglobin)

Hemolytic anemias caused by extraerythrocytic factors*

A. Extracorporeal factors
1. Isoantibodies due to ABO or Rh incompatibility (blood-typing and cross-matching)
2. Chemical agents and drugs such as phenylhydrazine, benzene, and lead (peripheral smear for lead)
3. Infectious agents such as malaria (malaria parasites on thick smear)
4. Physical agents such as aortic valve disease
5. Certain animal poisons such as snake and brown spider venoms

---

*The tests in parentheses are the diagnostic tests for each type of hemolytic anemia.

B. Conditions developing within the body
1. Idiopathic acquired hemolytic anemias (Coombs positive)
2. Secondary hemolytic anemias (Coombs negative) such as those associated with sarcoidosis (node biopsy and Kveim test), liver disease (liver function tests), Hodgkin's disease (node biopsy), disseminated lupus erythematosus (antinuclear antibodies), renal cortical necrosis (renal sediment and renal function tests), and thrombotic thrombocytopenic purpura (bone marrow and peripheral smear)

CHAPTER 10

Diagnostic tests for neurologic disorders

ANATOMY AND PHYSIOLOGY

The brain consists of three major parts: the cerebrum, the cerebellum, and the brainstem. The cerebrum is the largest division and is divided into two hemispheres, each of which has five lobes. The *cerebrum* is the highest integrative center of the nervous system and is responsible for sensation, perception, memory, consciousness, judgment, and will. The *cerebellum* is located just below the posterior portion of the cerebrum and functions in the control of skeletal muscles. The *brain stem* is composed of the midbrain, pons, and medulla oblongata, which connects the brain with the spinal cord and controls breathing, heart rate, and blood pressure.

The three meninges or membranes that envelop the brain and spinal cord are the *dura mater, arachnoid mater,* and *pia mater* (Fig. 10-2). Their names imply their qualities: the dura is the strong, tough outer layer; the arachnoid is a delicate layer between the dura mater and the pia mater; and the pia adheres to the brain surface like a delicate skin and contains blood vessels.

A potential space called the *subdural space* lies between the dura mater and the arachnoid mater. Between the arachnoid mater and the pia mater lies an actual space filled with cerebrospinal fluid called the *subarachnoid space*.

The *skull* is rigid and unyielding, and has very little space for anything but the brain. The skull can expand to accommodate hemorrhage, tumors, or fluid until a person is 12 or 13 years of age, when the skull sutures close. After this age anything in the skull taking up space pushes the brain down into the foramen magnum, the largest bony foramen in the skull. The foramen magnum lies at the lowest part of the skull and encircles the brain stem. Pressure from above pushes the brain down and the brain stem, with small cerebellar tonsils on each side, becomes impacted in the foramen magnum. This is a very critical anatomic area because the brain stem is involved with consciousness, control of blood pressure, heart rate, and respiration. If the brain stem does become impacted in the foramen magnum, it results in Cheyne-Stokes respirations, erratic breathing patterns, abnormal pupillary responses, and impairment of consciousness.

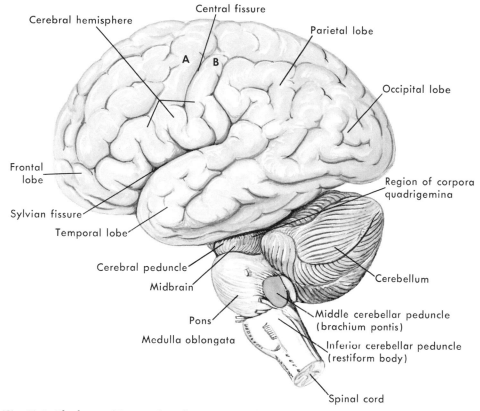

Cerebral hemisphere

Central fissure

Parietal lobe

A B

Occipital lobe

Frontal lobe

Region of corpora quadrigemina

Sylvian fissure

Temporal lobe

Cerebral peduncle

Midbrain

Cerebellum

Pons

Middle cerebellar peduncle (brachium pontis)

Medulla oblongata

Inferior cerebellar peduncle (restiform body)

Spinal cord

Fig. 10-1. The brain. (From Schottelius, B. A., and Schottelius, D. D.: Textbook of physiology, ed. 17, St. Louis, 1973, The C. V. Mosby Co.)

A second critical anatomic area is at the midbrain above the pons, where a sharp edge of dura separates the posterior fossa from the rest of the skull, dividing it into two compartments. This sharp edge of dura is positioned next to the midbrain on either side. If there is pressure on one side from a tumor, intracerebral hemorrhage, or the like, this uncus can be pushed down against the brain stem to the point where the brain stem is confined and held by the sharp edge of the dura. The third nerve comes out of the brain stem and travels in this area. The uncus can catch the third nerve, causing a dilated pupil on that side, or it can push the brain stem over to catch the third nerve on the other side, causing a dilated pupil on the other side.

LABORATORY TESTS IN BRAIN DISORDERS

In neurology the diagnosis and evaluation of the patient is usually much more dependent on the history and physical examination and expertise of the examiner in the interview than on laboratory tests. However, there are some laboratory tests that are valuable in evaluating and diagnosing neurologic conditions.

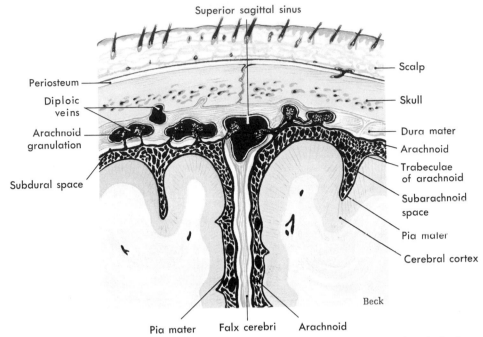

Fig. 10-2. The meninges of the brain as seen in coronal section through the skull. (From Anthony, C. P., and Kolthoff, N. J.: Textbook of anatomy and physiology, ed. 9, St. Louis, 1975, The C. V. Mosby Co.)

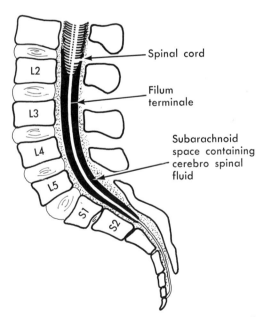

Fig. 10-3. The end of the spinal cord (lumbar vertebra 1-2).

The cerebrospinal fluid (CSF)

The cerebrospinal fluid (CSF) is the part of the central nervous system (CNS) that is most accessible to the clinician. The CSF is secreted by the cerebral vessels and the choroid plexuses, a cauliflower-like growth of blood vessels projecting into the lateral third and fourth ventricles of the brain. This fluid is continually secreted from the choroid plexus to pass into the fourth ventricle and from there into the subarachnoid cistern, where it diffuses over and around the brain and spinal cord. Although the spinal cord ends at the second lumbar vertebra, the subarachnoid space with its CSF extends to the second sacral vertebra.

The brain floats in CSF and is thus protected when the head receives a blow. Without the protection of the spinal fluid and meninges, the brain would probably be unable to withstand even the minor traumas of everyday living.

The spinal fluid is obtained through two sources: lumbar puncture and cisternal puncture. Cisternal puncture should not be performed by the inexperienced. However, lumbar puncture is a relatively harmless procedure and is easily done with some expertise.

Spinal taps should be done in any case of unexplained fever in which headaches are present and certainly when neck stiffness is present. It is indicated in most cases of suspected cerebral hemorrhage, with a few exceptions. If a thorough examination of the optic fundi reveals increased intracranial pressure, the spinal tap should be done with extreme caution, if indicated. If very high pressure is present in the head with the brain stem just about to wedge down into the foramen magnum, the release of fluid from the spinal canal will push the cerebellar tonsils along the brain stem, causing impaction in the foramen magnum and sudden death.

Procedure for spinal tap

The spinal tap is usually performed with an 18 gauge needle introduced between the fourth and fifth lumbar vertebrae or between the fifth lumbar and first sacral vertebrae. The opening and closing pressures can then be measured and the Queckenstedt test can be performed at the same time. In this test, pressure is placed on the external jugular veins while the spinal needle is connected to a manometer. If the fluid level rises and falls promptly with pressure on the jugulars and release of that pressure, there is no blockage of the free flow of CSF in the spinal column.

The Queckenstedt test should be done when the pathology is suspected to be in the spinal canal and not in the cranium. If there is pressure in the cranium, it is increased with this maneuver, and the brain stem may be pushed into the foramen magnum.

Gross appearance of spinal fluid

Blood. Blood in the spinal fluid may mean one of two things: either the tap was a bloody tap or intracranial hemorrhage might be indicated. The tap may be bloody because the spinal puncture is a blind procedure and a small vein or a venous plexus covering the spinal cord can be hit easily.

There are a few things that will help in differentiating between the two. Crenated red cells (a red blood cell that shows a scalloped border) are an indication that the hemorrhage is longer-standing than would be expected from a bloody tap. Also, the accidental bloody tap usually clears up after the initial bloody fluid and the fluid becomes relatively clear. If the tap is atraumatic but the fluid is bloody, subarachnoid hemorrhage is certain. Clear fluid helps in eliminating the possibility of intracranial hemorrhage and is helpful in the diagnosis of infections. If there is purulent infection then the test is not valid for protein and other determinations because the results will be obviously elevated.

Color. The normal CSF is a water-clear fluid. A xanthochromic (somewhat gold) fluid usually indicates the presence of either old blood or extreme elevation of protein in the central nervous system.

Turbidity indicates increased white and red cells as well as increased protein, in which case some kind of infectious process should be suspected.

If the CSF is frankly purulent, it is an indication of purulent meningitis and meningoencephalitis.

Microscopic examination of the CSF

The microscopic examination should be performed immediately after the CSF specimen is obtained. The specimen should be stained for both gram and acid-fast bacilli, and an indirect india ink stain for some specific fungi should be done. Normal values are found in Appendix A.

The cell count and differential. In a clear fluid a slight elevation of lymphocytes with slight protein elevation and a normal blood sugar level usually indicates an aseptic type of meningitis that may be viral or caused by a collagen disease.

An elevation of cells in proportion to the protein elevation suggests poliomyelitis. In Guillain-Barré syndrome, a proportional dissociation between decreased cells and increased protein is present, the so-called albuminocellular dissociation.

Protein elevation is also encountered in almost all serious pathologic conditions of the CNS. However, it should be noted that sometimes total protein may not be elevated in certain conditions (multiple sclerosis) when, qualitatively, immuno-electrophoresis may reveal abnormal proteins in 50% of the cases.

If the patient is suspected of having a CNS disease but yet does not have an elevated protein, a relatively benign condition is indicated.

Cultures of the CSF

When the CSF is purulent it is imperative to perform a culture. The patient's life may depend upon an accurate determination of the organism and its sensitivity. Cultures are usually done for aerobic and anaerobic microorganisms, acid-fast organisms, and fungi.

Sugar in the CSF

Normally the sugar in CSF is somewhat less than in blood, 45-75 mg/100 ml in the fasting adult.

Clinically, the sugar content in the CSF is important when it is low. Decreased sugar with apparently purulent CSF is typical of purulent meningitis, such as meningococcal meningitis, *Haemophilus influenzae* meningitis, or any bacterial meningitis. Viral meningitis is characterized by an elevated cell level and normal sugar level.

The sugar determination also becomes important when differentiating between viral meningitis and tubercular meningitis. Tubercular meningitis is characterized by decreased CSF sugar but viral meningitis is not. Both diseases may be similar in protein level and cytologic picture, making the CSF sugar the sole differentiating factor.

A simultaneous determination of serum blood sugar and CSF sugar should be obtained because, to be significant, the CSF sugar should be lower than two thirds of the blood sugar. There is a direct relationship between elevated blood sugar and elevated CSF sugar, since the composition of the CSF depends on filtration and diffusion from the blood.

Cytology

In suspected neoplasm (primary or metastatic), cytologic examination of the CSF may aid in the diagnosis of the malignancy.

VDRL (Venereal Disease Research Laboratories)

The VDRL test should be performed on the CSF in cases of suspected CNS syphillis particularly if a positive serology is to be evaluated in view of a negative history and a tertiary CNS syphilis is to be ruled out.

Radiologic examination of the skull and spinal column

Other accessible organs in evaluating the CNS are the skull and spinal column as seen on x-ray films.

X-ray film of the skull

This test requires the cooperation of the patient and is performed to verify fractures, abnormal calcification of a tumor, blood clots, or unilateral tumors.

X-ray films will reveal fractures when there has been trauma. When a neoplasm is suspected, particularly a multiple myeloma, x-ray films may be diagnostic. Calcification is normal in the pincal gland, which is located between the two halves of the thalamus. It can be determined if the gland is pushed to one side or not if it can be visualized on x-ray films. It should be exactly in the center of the two hemispheres of the brain. This is reliable information for determining the presence of a unilateral tumor or blood clot and intracranial calcification seen particularly in toxoplasmosis.

X-ray films of the spinal column

Sometimes pain in the extremities, or lumbar or thoracic regions can be detected by x-ray examination of the spinal column. Intervertebral disc involvement and encroachment and narrowing of the intervertebral disc and foramina can also be seen sometimes.

Brain scan

A brain scan requires a cooperative patient and is often performed as a diagnostic test because it is relatively atraumatic and should therefore precede more invasive methods.

This test depends on changes in the permeability of brain capillaries. Embryologically, brain tissue is skin and therefore, like skin, is a barrier tissue. There is, then, a blood-brain barrier that can be broken down by pathology such as a tumor, abscess, hemorrhage, focal injury, gunshot wound, and subdural hematoma. The radioisotopes that have been injected will concentrate in the involved area of the brain.

This test is very helpful in a patient who has suffered a recent stroke. Often a patient has a sudden hemiparesis or sudden speech deficit and one must determine whether it is caused by a stroke or a tumor. If a brain scan, taken in the first day or two after the impairment, is normal, it is good evidence that the impairment is a result of a stroke and not of a tumor or hemorrhage. Not much breakdown of brain tissue occurs until the third or fourth day following a stroke.

Electroencephalogram (EEG)

An electroencephalogram requires the cooperation of the patient and is performed to reveal focal abnormalities. The two halves of the brain are electrically identical in their function. Therefore, the left and right EEG patterns should be identical. Spike discharges in one area indicate a focal abnormality. Generalized slowing in the EEG waves indicates pressure that is causing diffuse problems in both hemispheres. This test is abnormal in 75% of patients with seizures, tumors, and subdural hematomas.

Electroencephalography is used to document focal epileptic lesions. However, there is a certain false negative in the EEG documentation of patients with chronic epilepsy.

In identifying a possible space-occupying lesion a normal EEG with a normal brain scan almost excludes a supratentorial brain tumor.

In cerebral vascular disease the EEG sometimes helps in the differential diagnosis between a tumor and an infarct.

In brain injury concussions the EEG helps in differentiating diffuse lesions from focal lesions.

Lastly, the EEG is becoming more and more important in defining cerebral death, particularly for medicolegal reasons in organ transplantation programs.

Sleeping electroencephalogram

This test is requested when the routine waking electroencephalogram is normal and yet a seizure or tumor is still suspected. The electrical rhythms of the brain are more unstable during sleep, when the pattern changes markedly. Abnormalities can sometimes be seen during sleep that cannot be seen when the patient is awake. A sleeping and waking EEG are always performed on patients who only have seizures during sleep. A sleeping EEG may occasionally show an abnormality in a situation in which a tumor is suspected and a diagnosis cannot be confirmed.

Echoencephalogram

This test does not require the cooperation of the patient. It is, therefore, a useful test for agitated patients.

The echoencephalogram is obtained by placing a titanium dioxide crystal at the head of the patient. This crystal emits a very high frequency sound wave that is echoed back when it hits an interface. Because sound travels at different rates through different densities, a change in density is recorded as a blip on the oscilloscope. The distance from the skull to the third ventricle of the brain is then measured on each side. Since the third ventricle should be in the exact center of the brain, it is evident immediately from this test if there is anything displacing one side of the brain. Of course, if the displacement is equal on both sides of the brain the echoencephalogram will give a false normal, since the third ventricle will still be in the center.

Electromyogram (EMG)

An electromyogram is a graph of the electrical potentials generated in individual muscles, which are usually tested at rest with slight voluntary contraction and with maximal contraction. This is accomplished by inserting a sterile needle electrode into the muscle to be tested. The electrical activity generated by the conduction mechanism of skeletal muscles is then amplified and displayed on a cathode-ray oscilloscope.

The electromyogram determines the following: (1) muscle denervation, (2) the level or area or nerve injury, (3) the presence of intrinsic muscle disease (dystrophies and myopathies), and (4) the occurrence of reinnervation.

The electromyogram is indicated as an aid in: (1) the diagnosis and the differential diagnosis of a large group of neuromuscular disorders involving the lower motor neuron, (2) determining the management of peripheral nerve injuries, (3) differentiating the apparent paralysis of the malingerer or the patient with hysteria, and (4) planning patient rehabilitation programs.

Invasive neurologic studies

Invasive tests should be performed only when noninvasive techniques do not establish the diagnosis, when there is need for subsequent action, such as in carotid occlusive disease with ischemic episodes, or in brain tumor evaluation.

Cerebral angiography

This test is done by aortic arch studies with selected angiography or by injecting a dye through the carotid artery, either right or left, depending on where the symptoms lie.

Angiography carries with it a small risk of about 1% from stroke, allergic reaction to the dye, or shock. It is important in detecting tumors, abscesses, hemorrhage, and thrombosis.

Pneumoencephalogram

In this test air is injected into the spinal fluid space in the lumbar area. Since this spinal fluid space is connected to the fluid spaces in the cranium, some of the air bubbles up and fills these fluid spaces in the head. The ventricles of the brain can then be visualized on x-ray films. If the brain has been displaced by the ventricles it will be evident. This test is usually performed when there is suspicion of hydrocephalus, increase or decrease of ventricular size, or deformity or displacement of the cerebral ventricles.

Myelogram

This test is performed by injecting a contrast medium into the spinal fluid. An x-ray film is then taken in order to visualize lesions suspected of causing cord compression. These lesions may be secondary to discogenic disease or neoplastic disease of the spinal column.

CHAPTER 11

Serodiagnostic tests

Some of the more common serologic procedures are discussed in this chapter. These procedures are used in the differential diagnosis of a wide variety of diseases and, more recently, in identifying and quantitating antibodies and antigens.

SEROLOGIC METHODS
Agglutination tests

Antibodies are capable of clumping both antigen molecules and bacteria together. This process is called *agglutination*. Agglutination reactions can be performed on a slide or in a test tube by mixing the patient's serum with the specific antigen. The presence of agglutination or clumping is then observed.

Complement fixation tests

This test involves a more tedious procedure. Complement is a substance, found in normal serum, that produces lysis when it is combined with antigen-antibody complexes. The patient's serum is first incubated with the antigen to be tested and a specific amount of complement. If an antigen-antibody reaction takes place, the complement will "fix" to these complexes. Erythrocytes coated with antibodies are then added to the combination and lysis occurs if there is any free complement left in the serum. The failure of lysis to occur implies that all of the complement was used up in the first phase of the test, indicating the presence of the particular antibody for which the test was performed.

Fluorescent antibody methods

In this test antibody attachment to an antigen is identified under the fluorescent microscope through the use of a fluorescent dye. A microscope slide is used upon which the clinical material has been fixed and overlaid with a specific preparation of antibody conjugated to dye. An antigen-antibody reaction is noted if fluorescent microorganisms are seen.

LABORATORY TESTS IN THE CLINICAL SETTING
Serodiagnosis of syphilis

Syphilis, a chronic systemic infection, is caused by the spirochete *Treponema pallidum* and is usually sexually transmitted.

Laboratory tests

The serodiagnosis of syphilis is based on two tests: the VDRL test as a screening test and the FTA-ABS test as a confirmatory test.

The VDRL (Venereal Disease Research Laboratories) is more or less nonspecific and is used for routine screening in almost all hospitals. It depends on the complement fixation test and a nonspecific reagent.

The definitive test is the FTA-ABS procedure (fluorescent treponemal antibody absorption test), which evolved after the introduction of the TPI (*Treponema pallidum* immobilization test), which is no longer performed routinely. In the FTA-ABS test the nonspecific antibodies are first removed from the patient's serum. The presence of specific antibodies is then demonstrated by the addition of the Nicols strain of *Treponema pallidum*, which makes the test highly specific.

Serodiagnosis of Salmonella

There are more than 1400 different serologic *Salmonella* types. The demonstration of serum antibodies is mainly helpful in the diagnosis of the typhoidal (*Salmonella typhi*) and septicemic forms.

Laboratory tests

Salmonella serum agglutinins in thyphoid fever were first demonstrated by the Widal test. Three antigens used in *Salmonella* serum serology are O antigen, H antigen, and Vi antigen.

Titers of O agglutinins are elevated by the end of the first week in 50% of patients with *Salmonella* disease. By the fourth week 90% to 95% of patients show an elevated titer.

Titers of H agglutinins rise slowly or not at all, peak later, may remain elevated for a few years, and are, therefore, not as reliable an indicator of *Salmonella* infections as are the O agglutinins.

The Vi agglutinins may be elevated when the O and H agglutinins are not elevated and are used, therefore, in suspected *Salmonella* carriers with negative O and H agglutinin titers.

In interpreting these tests, the patient's history should be considered since both O and H agglutinin titers can be elevated if the patient has been immunized or has come from an endemic area.

Serodiagnosis of Brucella

The *Brucella* microorganisms cause brucellosis (undulant fever), which may be either acute or chronic. They are transmitted to humans from animals, particularly goats (*B. melitensis*), hogs (*B. suis*), and cattle (*B. abortus*).

Laboratory tests

An agglutination test is used in the diagnosis of this disease, using a suspension of *Brucella abortus.* In acute brucellosis the titer begins to rise during the second week of the disease, peaking between the third and sixth weeks. In chronic brucellosis, an elevated agglutination titer may not be demonstrable without the use of anti-human globulin (Coombs technique).

Serodiagnosis of tularemia

Tularemia (rabbit fever, deer fly fever, Ohara's disease) is transmitted to humans from animals by direct contact or through an insect host. The causative organism is *Pasteurella (Francisella) tularensis,* a gram-negative bacillus.

Laboratory tests

The agglutination test for this disease uses a suspension of the bacterium *Francisella tularensis.* In patients with tularemia, titers of 1:80 are reached during the second week of infection, rising to 1:640 + in two to three months and then falling. Since cross-reactions with *Brucella* and *Proteus* OX-19 can occur, both should be tested to make the diagnosis of tularemia.

Serodiagnosis of rickettsial diseases

The rickettsial diseases of humans are caused by the parasites from the family Rickettsiaceae, which enter through the skin or the respiratory tract following infection.

Laboratory tests

The diagnosis of several of the rickettsial diseases can be made by the use of isolated strains of *Proteus,* designated OX-19, OX-2 and OX-K, which have antigens similar to those of the rickettsia. The resulting reaction is called the Weil-Felix reaction, after the men who isolated the *Proteus.*

The OX-19 reaction is positive in typhus and Rocky Mountain spotted fever. The OX-2 reaction is positive in the other spotted fevers: boutonneuse tick fever, Siberian tick typhus, Queensland tick typhus, and rickettsialpox. The OX-K reaction is positive for scrub typhus. There are no tests for the rest of the rickettsiae, such as trench fever or Q fever.

NOTE: Most of the serologic tests that have been described are ordered as febrile agglutinins in cases of fever of unknown etiology. All of them are done automatically in most hospitals under the heading of febrile agglutinins.

Serodiagnosis of streptococcic infection

Streptococci are important and common bacterial pathogens, entering the body through inhalation.

Laboratory tests

The antibodies used to test for streptococcus block the enzymatic extracellular product of the streptococcic organism. The tests are, therefore, antigen-antibody reactions. They include antistreptolysin-O (ASO), which is used most often, antihyaluronidase (AH), antistreptokinase, antideoxyribonuclease B (anti-DNAase-B), and antidiphosphopyridine nucleotidase (anti-DPNase).

Streptolysin O is an enzyme that is produced by group A *Streptococcus* and demonstrates antigenic activity. The antistreptolysin-O (ASO) titer is elevated in 80% of patients with nonsuppurative complications of streptococcic infections such as acute rheumatic fever and acute glomerulonephritis. It is elevated in 60% of patients with uncomplicated streptococcal disease, except in streptococcic pyoderma, in which only 25% of persons have an elevated ASO titer, although acute glomenulonephritis may also be present.

Hyaluronidase is another enzyme produced by group A *Streptococcus.* Antihyaluronidase (AH) used in combination with ASO increases the accuracy, and 90% of persons with streptococcic respiratory infection show an elevated titer to at least one of the two antigens. The titer of AH rises in the second week after infection and falls in three to five weeks.

Streptococcic deoxyribonuclease (DNA) (streptodornase) is the antigen used to demonstrate streptococcic pyoderma. The isoenzyme *anti-DNAase-B* has the most consistent antigen reaction.

Streptococcus MG is normally found in the upper respiratory tract of many persons. *Streptococcus MG* agglutinin titers rise in 45% to 50% of patients with clinical primary atypical pneumonia. This test correlates in most of these cases with an elevation of cold agglutinins.

Cold agglutinins, present in low titer in healthy persons, cause agglutination of red cells at 0° to 5° C. Generally, approximately 50% to 80% of patients with atypical pneumonia have elevated cold agglutinins secondary to mycoplasmal pneumonia, and the cold agglutinins present in the serum may cause hemolytic anemia. The rest of the atypical pneumonias are due to influenza A, influenza B, and parainfluenza viruses.

Autoantibodies in thyroid disease, rheumatoid arthritis, and systemic lupus erythematosus

Autoantibodies are produced by the body against one or more of its own tissue antigens, causing an antigen-antibody reaction with subsequent precipitation of the immune complexes on the blood vessels of multiple organs or production of injurious substances.

Thyroid disease

Several antibodies to tissue antigens are present in thyroid disease, including the following:
1. Thyroglobulin, found in 80% of patients with Hashimoto's thyroiditis
2. Cytoplasmic antigens
3. The colloid of thyroid follicles, demonstrated by fluorescent absorption technique
4. LATS (long-acting thyroid stimulator), the immunoglobulin found in 60% to 70% of patients with Graves' disease and appearing to react with the cell wall of the

thyroid epithelial cells, possibly at the site at which TSH attaches; it is found in the serum of patients with thyrotoxicosis, particularly if pretibial myxedema or exophthalmos is present.

The rheumatoid factor

Rheumatoid arthritis is a chronic systemic disease of unknown etiology that produces a globulin (19S or IgM immunoglobulin) in the serum of affected patients. The globulin, known as the rheumatoid factor reacts with the antigen, gamma G immunoglobulin, forming 22S globulin complex, suggesting that the rheumatoid factor in vivo reacts with IgG or IgM to form the immune complex. The immune complex, then, is the combination of IgM and IgG, IgG being the antigen and IgM the antibody produced against it.

In different groups of patients with clinical rheumatoid arthritis the ability to demonstrate the rheumatoid factor varies from 50% to 95%, with the higher percentile among patients with advanced disease and classical physical signs. If the patient has atypical signs or if the disease is of recent onset, the rheumatoid factor may be demonstrable in only 50% to 60% of the cases. If the rheumatoid arthritis is psoriatic arthritis or juvenile rheumatoid arthritis, as few as 10% to 25% of the patients will have the rheumatoid factor, probably indicating the difference between the diseases rather than the similarities.

Systemic lupus erythematosus

In the diagnosis of systemic lupus erythematosus (SLE), the first test to be described was the LE cell phenomenon, which is the demonstration of antinuclear antibodies in SLE. The antibody is produced against the nuclear part of the white blood cell (antigens). The LE cell is a large neutrophil that contains the products of this reaction plus complement and the damaged material ingested by the neutrophils.

More specific than the LE cell phenomenon is the test for antinuclear antibodies, the presence of which is the distinguishing characteristic of SLE. Antinuclear antibodies are gamma globulins that react to nuclear antigens, such as nuclear proteins, deoxyribonucleic acid (DNA), histones, and soluble antigens. Also, some patients with SLE have antibodies against ribonucleic acid (RNA), cytosomes, lysomes, and other cytoplasmic constituents. These antinuclear factors usually belong to more than one immunoglobulin class: IgG is seen in 96% of patients, IgM in 80%, and IgA in 50%. In patients with anti-DNA antibodies, the antibodies are usually of the IgG subclass, which binds complement. Many of these antibodies persist even after the disease is quiescent.

Complement fixation accompanies a reaction between the antigen and the antibody. Thus, in the beginning of the acute disease state, the complement level, particularly the C_3 fraction, significantly drops. In other words, the antigen (DNA or RNA) plus the antibody plus the complement is the immune complex. The diseases produced are called immune complex diseases. As mentioned on p. 180 this immune complex produces disease by depositing itself in various vessels, causing vasculitis and glomerulonephritis, which are the important aspects of lupus erythematosus.

From a diagnostic point of view, the most important tests are those demonstrating antinuclear antibodies and a sudden drop in complement, the latter heralding the initiation of an acute episode of SLE.

The SLE phenomena and an increase of antinuclear antibodies in the serum are associated with certain types of prolonged medication, such as antihypertensives (hydralazine), anticonvulsants, procainamide, and isoniazid. However, when these medications are discontinued ANA in the serum becomes undetectable.

Serodiagnosis of parasitic disease

In parasitic diseases, serologic procedures are used if the parasites or their ova cannot be identified in feces, blood, or body tissues.

Laboratory tests

Serologic tests are available for the following diseases: trichinosis, amebiasis, toxoplasmosis, schistosomiasis, and echinoccocus cysts. The most useful of all of these tests is the one employed for the diagnosis of echinoccal cysts, since other methods of diagnosis, such as aspiration or biopsy, are extremely difficult and can be dangerous.

In acute amebiasis biopsy is not as helpful in the diagnosis as is seeing the ameba in the stool. In schistosomiasis the best diagnostic test is probably a rectal biopsy, since a positive serology is not necessarily diagnostic and a negative test does not necessarily indicate the absence of the disease. Up to 15% of noninfected persons have a positive test, while approximately 75% of persons with the disease have a positive test.

Serodiagnosis of infectious mononucleosis

Infectious mononucleosis is an acute infectious disease of the reticuloendothelial tissues caused by the Epstein-Barr virus. The serum of these patients contains, in high titer, antibodies (heterophil antibodies) that agglutinate sheep and horse red blood cells. Several tests are available for the demonstration of antisheep and antihorse agglutinins.

Laboratory tests

Presumptive test. Antisheep and antihorse agglutinins are present, in titers of less than 112, in the serum of most people. When the clinical and hematologic findings are characteristic of infectious mononucleosis, a titer of 224 or more is considered diagnostic. The titer may also be elevated in serum disease and in a variety of infections.

Differential test. Differentiation is accomplished through absorption techniques using guinea pig or horse kidney and beef red blood cells. The antisheep agglutinins in the serum of patients with serum disease and other infections are absorbed in a suspension of guinea pig or horse kidney. This does not occur with the serum of patients with infectious mononucleosis. Conversely, the antisheep agglutinins in the serum of patients with infectious mononucleosis is absorbed by beef red blood cells. This does not occur with the other infections.

   The spot test. This is a slide test in which the patient's serum is mixed with guinea pig kidney on one spot of the slide and with beef red blood cells on another. Horse red blood cells are then added to each spot. In infectious mononucleosis agglutination occurs with the guinea pig kidney suspension. The agglutination with the beef red blood cells is less than the guinea pig kidney.

Appendices

APPENDIX A

Tables of normal values

Many of the normal values are based on the experience in the Department of Pathology, Mount Sinai Hospital, Chicago, Illinois, and the Division of Clinical Pathology, State University Hospital, State University of New York, Syracuse, New York. Actual values may vary with different techniques or in different laboratories. Although only the more common tests are discussed in the text, others are included here for completeness.

ABBREVIATIONS USED IN TABLES

<	= less than	mIU	= milliInternational Unit
>	= greater than	mOsm	= milliosmole
dl	= 100 ml	mμ	= millimicron
gm	= gram	ng	= nanogram
IU	= International Unit	pg	= picogram
kg	= kilogram	μEq	= microequivalent
mEq	= milliequivalent	μg	= microgram
mg	= milligram	μIU	= microInternational Unit
ml	= milliliter	μl	= microliter
mM	= millimole	μU	= microunit
mm Hg	= millimeters of mercury		

Reproduced with permission from Davidsohn, I. and Henry, J. B. editors: Todd-Sanford Clinical diagnosis by laboratory methods, ed. 15, Philadelphia, 1974. W. B. Saunders Co.

Table A-1. Whole blood, serum, and plasma (chemistry)

Test	Material	Normal value	Special instructions
Acetoacetic acid			
Qualitative	Serum	Negative	
Quantitative	Serum	0.2-1.0 mg/dl	
Acetone			
Qualitative	Serum	Negative	
Quantitative	Serum	0.3-2.0 mg/dl	
Albumin, quantitative	Serum	3.2-4.5 gm/dl (salt fractionation) 3.2-5.6 gm/dl by electrophoresis 3.8-5.0 gm/dl by dye binding	
Alcohol	Serum or whole blood	Negative	
Aldolase	Serum	Adults: 3-8 Sibley-Lehninger U/dl at 37° C Children: Approximately 2 times adult levels Newborn: Approximately 4 times adult levels	
Alpha-amino acid nitrogen	Serum	3-6 mg/dl	
δ-Aminolevulinic acid	Serum	0.01-0.03 mg/dl	
Ammonia	Plasma	20-150 μg/dl (diffusion) 40-80 μg/dl (enzymatic method) 12-48 μg/dl (resin method)	Collect with sodium heparinate; specimen must be analyzed immediately
Amylase	Serum	60-160 Somogyi units/dl	
Argininosuccinic lyase	Serum	0-4 U/dl	
Arsenic	Whole blood	<3 μg/dl	
Ascorbic acid (vitamin C)	Plasma Whole blood	0.6-1.6 mg/dl 0.7-2.0 mg/dl	Analyze immediately
Barbiturates	Serum, plasma, or whole blood	Negative	
Base excess	Whole blood	Male: −3.3 to +1.2 Female: −2.4 to +2.3	
Base, total	Serum	145-160 mEq/L	
Bicarbonate	Plasma	21-28 mM/L	
Bile acids	Serum	0.3-3.0 mg/dl	
Bilirubin	Serum	Up to 0.3 mg/dl (direct or conjugated) 0.1-1.0 mg/dl (indirect or unconjugated) Total: 0.1-1.2 mg/dl Newborns total: 1-12 mg/dl	

Table A-1. Whole blood, serum, and plasma (chemistry)—cont'd

Test	Material	Normal value	Special instructions
Blood gases			
pH		7.38-7.44 arterial	
		7.36-7.41 venous	
Pco$_2$		35-40 mm Hg arterial	
		40-45 mm Hg venous	
Po$_2$		95-100 mm Hg arterial	
Bromide	Serum	0-5 mg/dl	
BSP (bromsulfonphthalein) (5 mg/kg)	Serum	<6% retention after 45 min	
Calcium	Serum	Ionized: 4.2-5.2 mg/dl 2.1-2.6 mEq/L or 50-58% of total Total: 9.0-10.6 mg/dl 4.5-5.3 mEq/L Infants: 11-13 mg/dl	
Carbon dioxide (CO$_2$ content)	Whole blood, arterial	19-24 mM/L	
	Plasma or serum, arterial	21-28 mM/L	
	Whole blood, venous	22-26 mM/L	
	Plasma or serum, venous	24-30 mM/L	
CO$_2$ combining power	Plasma or serum, venous	24-30 mM/L	
CO$_2$ partial pressure (Pco$_2$)	Whole blood, arterial	35-40 mm Hg	
	Whole blood, venous	40-45 mm Hg	
Carbonic acid	Whole blood, arterial	1.05-1.45 mM/L	
	Whole blood, venous	1.15-1.50 mM/L	
	Plasma, venous	1.02-1.38 mM/L	
Carboxyhemoglobin (carbon monoxide hemoglobin)	Whole blood	Suburban nonsmokers: <1.5% saturation of hemoglobin Smokers: 1.5-5.0% saturation Heavy smokers: 5.0-9.0% saturation	
Carotene, beta	Serum	40-200 μg/dl	
Cephalin cholesterol flocculation	Serum	Negative to 1+ after 24 hours 2+ or less after 48 hours	
Ceruloplasmin	Serum	23-50 mg/dl	
Chloride	Serum	95-103 mEq/L	
Cholesterol, total	Serum	150-250 mg/dl (varies with diet and age)	

Continued.

Table A-1. Whole blood, serum, and plasma (chemistry)—cont'd

Test	Material	Normal value	Special instructions
Cholesterol, esters	Serum	65-75% of total cholesterol	
Cholinesterase	Erythrocytes	0.65-1.00 pH units	
Pseudocholinesterase	Plasma	0.5-1.3 pH units 8-18 IU/L at 37° C	
Citric acid	Serum or plasma	1.7-3.0 mg/dl	
Congo red test	Serum or plasma	>60% after 1 hour	Severe reactions may occur if dye is injected twice; check patient's record
Copper	Serum or plasma	Male: 70-140 μg/dl Female: 85-155 μg/dl	
Cortisol	Plasma	8 A.M.-10 A.M.: 5-25 μg/dl 4 P.M.-6 P.M.: 2-18 μg/dl	
Creatine	Serum or plasma	Males: 0.2-0.6 mg/dl Females: 0.6-1.0 mg/dl	
Creatine phosphokinase (CPK)	Serum	Males: 55-170 U/L at 37° C Females: 30-135 U/L at 37° C	See Chapter 4
Creatinine	Serum or plasma	0.6-1.2 mg/dl	
Creatinine clearance (endogenous)	Serum or plasma and urine	Male: 123 + 16 ml/min Female: 97 ± 10 ml/min	
Cryoglobulins	Serum	Negative	Keep specimen at 37° C
Electrophoresis, protein	Serum	*percent* *gm/dl* Albumin 52-65 3.2-5.6 Alpha-1 2.5-5.0 0.1-0.4 Alpha-2 7.0-13.0 0.4-1.2 Beta 8.0-14.0 0.5-1.1 Gamma 12.0-22.0 0.5-1.6	
Fats, neutral	Serum or plasma	0-200 mg/dl	

Fatty acids
  Total
  Free
	
	Serum
	Plasma
		
		9-15 mM/L
		300-480 μEq/L	

Fibrinogen	Plasma	200-400 mg/dl	
Fluoride	Whole blood	<0.05 mg/dl	
Folate	Serum Erythrocytes	5-25 ng/ml (bioassay) 166-640 ng/ml (bioassay)	
Galactose	Whole blood	Adults: none Children: <20 mg/dl	
Gammaglobulin	Serum	0.5-1.6 gm/dl	

Table A-1. Whole blood, serum, and plasma (chemistry)—cont'd

Test	Material	Normal value	Special instructions
Globulins, total	Serum	2.3-3.5 gm/dl	
Glucose, fasting	Serum or plasma Whole blood	70-110 mg/dl 60-100 mg/dl	Collect with heparin-fluoride mixture
Glucose tolerance, oral	Serum or plasma	Fasting: 70-110 mg/dl 30 min: 30-60 mg/dl above fasting 60 min: 20-50 mg/dl above fasting 120 min: 5-15 mg/dl above fasting 180 min: fasting level or below	Collect with heparin-fluoride mixture
Glucose tolerance, IV	Serum or plasma	Fasting: 70-110 mg/dl 5 min: Maximum of 250 mg/dl 60 min: Significant decrease 120 min: Below 120 mg/dl 180 min: Fasting level	Collect with heparin-fluoride mixture
Glucose-6-phosphate dehydrogenase (G-6-PD)	Erythrocytes	250-500 units/10^9 cells 1200-2000 mIU/ml of packed erythrocytes	
γ-Glutamyl transpeptidase	Serum	2-39 U/L	
Glutathione	Whole blood	24-37 mg/dl	
Growth hormone	Serum	<10 ng/ml	
Guanase	Serum	<3 nM/ml/min	
Haptoglobin	Serum	100-200 mg/dl as hemoglobin binding capacity	
Hemoglobin	Serum or plasma	Qualitative: Negative Quantitative: 0.5-5.0 mg/dl	
Hemoglobin	Whole blood	Female: 12.0-16.0 gm/dl Male: 13.5-18.0 gm/dl	
Hemoglobin A_2	Whole blood	1.5-3.5% of total hemoglobin	
α-Hydroxybutyric dehydrogenase	Serum	140-350 U/ml	
17-Hydroxycorticosteroids	Plasma	Male: 7-19 μg/dl Female: 9-21 μg/dl After 25 USP units of ACTH IM: 35-55 μg/dl	Perform test immediately or freeze plasma
Immunoglobulins IgG IgA IgM IgD IgE	Serum	 800-1600 mg/dl 50-250 mg/dl 40-120 mg/dl 0.5-3.0 mg/dl 0.01-0.04 mg/dl	

Continued.

Table A-1. Whole blood, serum, and plasma (chemistry)—cont'd

Test	Material	Normal value	Special instructions
Insulin	Plasma	11-240 μIU/ml (bioassay) 4-24 μU/ml (radioimmunoassay)	
Insulin tolerance	Serum	Fasting: Glucose of 70-110 mg/dl 30 min : Fall to 50% of fasting level 90 min : Fasting level	Collect with heparin- fluoride mixture
Iodine Butanol extraction (BEI) Protein bound (PBI)	Serum Serum	3.5-6.5 μg/dl 4.0-8.0 μg/dl	Test not reliable if iodine- containing drugs or radiographic contrast media were given prior to test
Iron, total Iron-binding capacity Iron saturation, percent	Serum Serum Serum	50-150 μg/dl 250-450 μg/dl 20-55%	Hemolysis must be avoided
Isocitric dehydrogenase	Serum	50-250 U/ml	
Ketone bodies	Serum	Negative	
17-Ketosteroids	Plasma	25-125 μg/dl	
Lactic acid	Whole blood, venous Whole blood, arterial	5-20 mg/dl 3-7 mg/dl	Draw without stasis
Lactate dehydrogenase (LDH)	Serum	80-120 Wacker units 150-450 Wroblewski units 71-207 IU/L	See Chapter 4
Lactate dehydrogenase isoenzymes	Serum	Anode: LDH_1 17-27% LDH_2 27-37% LDH_3 18-25% LDH_4 3-8% Cathode: LDH_5 0-5%	
Lactate dehydrogenase (heat stable)	Serum	30-60% of total	
Lactose tolerance	Serum	Serum glucose changes are similar to those seen in a glucose tolerance test	
Lead	Whole blood	0-50 μg/dl	
Leucine aminopept. lase (LAP)	Serum	Male: 80-200 Goldbarg- Rutenburg units/ml Female: 75-185 Goldbarg- Rutenburg units/ml	

Table A-1. Whole blood, serum, and plasma (chemistry)—cont'd

Test	Material	Normal value	Special instructions
Lipase	Serum	0-1.5 Cherry-Crandall U/ml 14-280 mIU/ml	
Lipids Total Cholesterol Triglycerides Phospholipids Fatty acids Neutral fat Phospholipid phosphorus	Serum	 400-800 mg/dl 150-250 mg/dl 10-190 mg/dl 150-380 mg/dl 9.0-15.0 mM/L 0-200 mg/dl 8.0-11.0 mg/dl	
Lithium	Serum	Negative Therapeutic level: 0.5-1.5 mEq/L	
Long-acting thyroid- stimulating hormone (LATS)	Serum	None	
Luteinizing hormone (LH)	Plasma	Male: <11 mIU/ml Female: midcycle peak >3 times baseline value Premenopausal: <25 mIU/ml Postmenopausal: >25 mIU/ml	
Macroglobulins, total	Serum	70-430 mg/dl	
Magnesium	Serum	1.5-2.5 mEq/L 1.8-3.0 mg/dl	
Methemoglobin	Whole blood	0-0.24 gm/dl 0.4-1.5% of total hemoglobin	
Mucoprotein	Serum	80-200 mg/dl	
Nonprotein nitrogen (NPN)	Serum or plasma Whole blood	20-35 mg/dl 25-50 mg/dl	
5′ Nucleotidase	Serum	0-1.6 units	
Ornithine carbamyl transferase (OCT)	Serum	8-20 mIU/ml	
Osmolality	Serum	280-295 mOsm/L	
Oxygen Pressure (PO_2)	Whole blood, arterial	95-100 mm Hg	
Content	Whole blood, arterial	15-23 vol %	
Saturation	Whole blood, arterial	94-100%	
pH	Whole blood, arterial	7.38-7.44	
	Whole blood, venous	7.36-7.41	
	Serum or plasma, venous	7.35-7.45	

Continued.

Table A-1. Whole blood, serum, and plasma (chemistry)—cont'd

Test	Material	Normal value	Special instructions
Phenylalanine	Serum	Adults: <3.0 mg/dl Newborns (term): 1.2-3.5 mg/dl	
Phosphatase, acid, total	Serum	0-1.1 U/ml (Bodansky) 1-4 U/ml (King-Armstrong) 0.13-0.63 U/ml (Bessey-Lowry) 1.4-5.5 U/ml (Gutman-Gutman) 0-0.56 U/ml (Roy) 0-6.0 U/ml (Shinowara-Jones-Reinhart)	Hemolysis must be avoided; perform test without delay or freeze specimen
Phosphatase, alkaline, total	Serum	Adults: 1.5-4.5 U/dl (Bodansky) 4-13 U/dl (King-Armstrong) 0.8-2.3 U/ml (Bessey-Lowry) 15-35 U/ml (Shinowara-Jones-Reinhart) Children: 5.0-14.0 U/dl (Bodansky) 3.4- 9.0 U/ml (Bessey-Lowry) 15-30 U/dl (King-Armstrong)	
Phospholipid phosphorus	Serum	8-11 mg/dl	
Phospholipids	Serum	150-380 mg/dl	
Phosphorus, inorganic	Serum	Adults: 1.8-2.6 mEq/L 3.0-4.5 mg/dl Children: 2.3-4.1 mEq/L 4.0-7.0 mg/dl	Separate cells from serum promptly
Potassium	Plasma	3.8-5.0 mEq/L	
Proteins Total Albumin Globulin	Serum	 6.0-7.8 gm/dl 3.2-4.5 gm/dl 2.3-3.5 gm/dl	
Protein fractionation	Serum		
Protoporphyrin	Erythrocytes	15-50 μg/dl	
Pyruvate	Whole blood	0.3-0.9 mg/dl	
Salicylates	Serum	Negative Therapeutic level: 20-25 mg/dl	
Sodium	Plasma	136-142 mEq/L	
Sulfate, inorganic	Serum	0.2-1.3 mEq/L 0.9-6.0 mg/dl as SO_4	Hemolysis must be avoided
Sulfhemoglobin	Whole blood	Negative	
Sulfonamides	Serum or whole blood	Negative	
Testosterone	Serum or plasma	Male: 400-1200 ng/dl Female: 30-120 ng/dl	

Table A-1. Whole blood, serum, and plasma (chemistry)—cont'd

Test	*Material*	*Normal value*	*Special instructions*
Thiocyanate	Serum	Negative	
Thymol flocculation	Serum	0-5 units	
Thyroid hormone tests	Serum	*Espressed as thyroxine* *Expressed as iodine*	
T_4 (by column)		5.0-11.0 μg/dl 3.2-7.2 μg/dl	
T_4 (by competitive binding Murphy-Pattee)		6.0-11.8 μg/dl 3.9-7.7 μg/dl	
Free T_4		0.9-2.3 ng/dl 0.6-1.5 ng/dl	
T_3 (resin uptake)		25-38 relative % uptake	
Thyroxine-binding globulin (TBG)		10-26 μg/dl (expressed as T_4 uptake)	
Transaminases			
GOT	Serum	8-33 U/ml	
GPT	Serum	1-36 U/ml	
Triglycerides	Serum	10-190 mg/dl	
Urea nitrogen	Serum	8-18 mg/dl	
Urea clearance	Serum and urine	Maximum clearance: 64-99 ml/min Standard clearance: 41-65 ml/min or more than 75% of normal clearance	
Uric acid	Serum	Male: 2.1-7.8 mg/dl Female: 2.0-6.4 mg/dl	
Vitamin A	Serum	15-60 μg/dl	
Vitamin A tolerance	Serum	Fasting: 15-60 μg/dl 3 hr. or 6 hr. after 5000 units vitamin A/kg: 200-600 μg/dl 24 hr: fasting values or slightly above	Administer 5000 units vitamin A in oil per kg body weight
Vitamin B_{12}	Serum	Male: 200-800 pg/ml Female: 100-650 pg/ml	
Unsaturated vitamin B_{12} binding capacity	Serum	1000-2000 pg/ml	
Vitamin C	Plasma	0.6-1.6 mg/dl	Collect with oxalate and analyze within 20 minutes
Xylose absorption	Serum	25-40 mg/dl between 1 and 2 hr; in malabsorption, maximum approximately 10 mg/dl Dose Adult: 25 gm D-xylose Children: 0.5 gm/kg D-xylose	For children administer 10 ml of a 5% solution of D-xylose per kg of body weight
Zinc	Serum	50-150 μg/dl	
Zinc sulfate turbidity	Serum	< 12 units	

Table A-2. Urine

Test	Type of specimen	Normal value	Special instructions
Acetoacetic acid	Random	Negative	
Acetone	Random	Negative	
Addis count	12-hr collection	WBC and epithelial cells: 1,800,000/12 hr RBC: 500,000/12 hr Hyaline casts: 0-5,000/12 hr	Rinse bottle with some neutral formalin; discard excess
Albumin			
Qualitative	Random	Negative	
Quantitative	24 hr	10-100 mg/24 hr	
Aldosterone	24 hr	2-26 μg/24 hr	Keep refrigerated
Alkapton bodies	Random	Negative	
Alpha-amino acid nitrogen	24 hr	100-290 mg/24 hr	
δ-Aminolevulinic acid	Random	Adult: 0.1-0.6 mg/dl Children: <0.5 mg/dl	
	24 hr	1.5-7.5 mg/24 hr	
Ammonia nitrogen	24 hr	20-70 mEq/24 hr 500-1200 mg/24 hr	Keep refrigerated
Amylase	2 hr	35-260 Somogyi units per hour	
Arsenic	24 hr	<50 μg/L	
Ascorbic acid	Random	1-7 mg/dl	
	24 hr	>50 mg/24 hr	
Bence Jones protein	Random	Negative	
Beryllium	24 hr	<0.05 μg/24 hr	
Bilirubin, qualitative	Random	Negative	
Blood, occult	Random	Negative	
Borate	24 hr	<2 mg/L	
Calcium			
Qualitative (Sulko-witch)	Random	1 + turbidity	Compare with standard
Quantitative	24 hr	Average diet: 100-250 mg/24 hr Low calcium diet: <150 mg/24 hr High calcium diet: 250-300 mg/24 hr	
Catecholamines	Random	0-14 μg/dl	
	24 hr	<100 μg/24 hr (varies with activity)	
Chloride	24 hr	110-250 mEq/24 hr	
Concentration test (Fishberg)	Random after fluid restriction	Specific gravity: >1.025 Osmolality: >850 mOsm/L	
Copper	24 hr	0-30 μg/24 hr	

Table A-2. Urine—cont'd

Test	Type of specimen	Normal value	Special instructions
Coproporphyrin	Random 24 hr	Adult: 3-20 μg/dl 50-160 μg/24 hr Children: 0-80 μg/24 hr	Use fresh specimen and do not expose to direct light; preserve 24-hr urine with 5 gm Na_2CO_3
Creatine	24 hr	Male: 0-40 mg/24 hr Female: 0-100 mg/24 hr Higher in children and during pregnancy	
Creatinine	24 hr	Male: 20-26 mg/kg/24 hr 1.0-2.0 gm/24 hr Female: 14-22 mg/kg/24 hr 0.8-1.8 gm/24 hr	
Cystine, qualitative	Random	Negative	
Cystine and cysteine	24 hr	10-100 mg/24 hr	
Diacetic acid	Random	Negative	
Epinephrine	24 hr	0-20 μg/24 hr	
Estrogens, total	24 hr	Male: 5-18 μg/24 hr Female Ovulation: 28-100 μg/24 hr Luteal peak: 22-105 μg/24 hr At menses: 4-25 μg/24 hr Pregnancy: up to 45,000 μg/24 hr Postmenopausal: 14-20 μg/24 hr	Keep refrigerated
Estrogens, Fractionated Estrone (E1) Estradiol (E2) Estriol (E3)	24 hr	Non-pregnant, mid-cycle 2-25 μg/24 hr 0-10 μg/24 hr 2-30 μg/24 hr	
Fat, qualitative	Random	Negative	
FIGLU (N-formi-minoglutamic acid)	24 hr	<3 mg/24 hr After 15 gm of L-histidine: 4 mg/8 hr	
Fluoride	24 hr	<1 mg/24 hr	
Follicle-stimulating hormone (FSH)	24 hr	Adult: 6-50 mouse uterine units/24 hr Prepubertal: <MUU/24 hr Post-menopausal: >MUU/24 hr	
Fructose	24 hr	30-65 mg/24 hr	
Glucose Qualitative Quantitative copper-reducing substances	Random 24 hr	Negative 0.5-1.5 gm/24 hr	

Continued.

Table A-2. Urine—cont'd

Test	Type of specimen	Normal value	Special instructions
Glucose—cont'd Quantitative—cont'd total sugars glucose		Average: 250 mg/24 hr Average: 130 mg/24 hr	
Gonadotropins, pituitary (FSH and LH)	24 hr	10-50 MUU/24 hr	
Hemoglobin	Random	Negative	
Homogentisic acid	Random	Negative	
Homovanillic acid (HVA)	24 hr	<15 mg/24 hr	
17-Hydroxycortico-steroids	24 hr	Male: 5.5-14.5 mg/24 hr Female: 4.9-12.9 mg/24 hr Lower in children After 25 USP units ACTH, IM: a 2- to 4-fold increase	Keep refrigerated
5-Hydroxyindole-acetic acid, qualitative	Random	Negative	Some muscle relaxants and tranquilizers interfere with test
5-HIAA, quantitative	24 hr	<9 mg/24 hr	
Indican	24 hr	10-20 mg/24 hr	
Ketone bodies	Random	Negative	Fresh, keep cool
17-Ketosteroids	24 hr	Male: 8-15 mg/24 hr Female: 6-11.5 mg/24 hr Children: 12-15 yr, 5-12 mg/24 hr; <12 yr, <5 mg/24 hr After 25 USP units ACTH, IM: 50-100% increase	Keep refrigerated;
Androsterone		Male: 2.0-5.0 mg/24 hr Female: 0.8-3.0 mg/24 hr	
Etiocholanolone		Male: 1.4-5.0 mg/24 hr Female: 0.8-4.0 mg/24 hr	
Dehydroepiandro-sterone		Male: 0.2-2.0 mg/24 hr Female: 0.2-1.8 mg/24 hr	
11-Ketoandro-sterone		Male: 0.2-1.0 mg/24 hr Female: 0.2-0.8 mg/24 hr	
11-Ketoetio-cholanolone		Male: 0.2-1.0 mg/24 hr Female: 0.2-0.8 mg/24 hr	
11-Hydroxyandro-sterone		Male: 0.1-0.8 mg/24 hr Female: 0.0-0.5 mg/24 hr	
11-Hydroxyetio-cholanolone		Male: 0.2-0.6 mg/24 hr Female: 0.1-1.1 mg/24 hr	

Table A-2. Urine—cont'd

Test	Type of specimen	Normal value	Special instructions
Lactose	24 hr	12-40 mg/24 hr	
Lead	24 hr	<100 μg/24 hr	
Magnesium	24 hr	6.0-8.5 mEq/24 hr	
Melanin, qualitative	Random	Negative	
3-Methoxy-4-hydroxy-mandelic acid (VMA)	24 hr	1.5-7.5 mg/24 hr (adults) 83 μg/kg/24 hr (infants)	No coffee or fruit two days prior to test
Mucin	24 hr	100-150 mg/24 hr	
Myoglobin			
Qualitative	Random	Negative	
Quantitative	24 hr	<1.5 mg/L	
Osmolality	Random	500-800 mOsm/L	May be lower or higher, depending on state of hydration
Pentoses	24 hr	2-5 mg/kg/24 hr	
pH	Random	4.6-8.0	
Phenolsulfonphthalein (PSP)	Urine, timed after 6 mg PSP IV		
15 min		20-50% dye excreted	
30 min		16-24% dye excreted	
60 min		9-17% dye excreted	
120 min		3-10% dye excreted	
Phenylpyruvic acid, qualitative	Random	Negative	
Phosphorus	Random	0.9-1.3 gm/24 hr	Varies with intake
Porphobilinogen			
Qualitative	Random	Negative	
Quantitative	24 hr	0-2.0 mg/24 hr	
Potassium	24 hr	40-80 mEq/24 hr	Varies with diet
Pregnancy tests	Concentrated morning specimen	Positive in normal pregnancies or with tumors producing chorionic gonadotropin	

Pregnanediol	24 hr	Male: 0-1 mg/24 hr
		Female: 1-8 mg/24 hr
		  Peak: 1 week after ovulation
		  Pregnancy: 60-100 mg/24 hr
		Children: Negative
			Keep refrigerated

Pregnanetriol	24 hr	Male: 1.0-2.0 mg/24 hr Female: 0.5-2.0 mg/24 hr Children: <0.5 mg/24 hr	Keep refrigerated

Continued.

Table A-2. Urine—cont'd

Test	Type of specimen	Normal value	Special instructions
Protein			
Qualitative	Random	Negative	
Quantitative	24 hr	10-100 mg/24 hr	
Reducing substances, total	24 hr	0.5-1.5 mg/24 hr	
Sodium	24 hr	80-180 mEq/24 hr	Varies with dietary ingestion of salt
Solids, total	24 hr	55-70 gm/24 hr Decreases with age to 30 gm/24 hr	
Specific gravity	Random	1.016-1.022 (normal fluid intake) 1.001-1.035 (range)	
Sugars (excluding glucose)	Random	Negative	
Titrable acidity	24 hr	20-50 mEq/24 hr	Collect with toluene
Urea nitrogen	24 hr	6-17 gm/24 hr	
Uric acid	24 hr	250-750 mg/24 hr	Varies with diet
Urobilinogen	2 hr 24 hr	0.3-1.0 Ehrlich units 0.05-2.5 mg/24 hr or 0.5-4.0 Ehrlich units/24 hr	
Uropepsin	Random 24 hr	15-45 units/hr 1500-5000 units/24 hr	
Uroporphyrins			
Qualitative	Random	Negative	
Quantitative	24 hr	10-30 μg/24 hr	
Vanillylmandelic acid (VMA)	24 hr	1.5-7.5 mg/24 hr	
Volume, total	24 hr	600-1600 ml/24 hr	
Zinc	24 hr	0.15-1.2 mg/24 hr	

Table A-3. Gastric fluid

Test	Normal value
Fasting residual volume	20-100 ml
pH	<2.0
Basal acid output (BAO)	0-6 mEq/hr
Maximal acid output (MAO) after histamine stimulation	5-40 mEq/h4
BAO/MAO ratio	<0.4

Table A-4. Hematology

Test	Normal value		
Hemoglobin A$_2$	1.5-3.5%		
Hemoglobin F	<2%		

Osmotic fragility

% Na Cl	% Lysis (fresh)	% Lysis (after 24-hr incubation at 37° C)
0.20	97-100	95-100
0.30	90-99	85-100
0.35	50-95	75-100
0.40	5-45	65-100
0.45	0-6	55-95
0.50	0	40-85
0.55		15-70
0.60		0-40
0.65		0-10
0.70		0-5
0.75		0

Test	Normal value
Platelet count	150,000-400,000/μl
Reticulocyte count	0.5-1.5% 25,000-75,000 cells/μl
Sedimentation rate (ESR) (Westergren)	Men under 50 yr: <15 mm/h4 Men over 50 yr: <20 mm/hr Women under 50 yr: <20 mm/hr Women over 50 yr: <30 mm/hr
Viscosity	1.4-1.8 times water
Complete blood count (CBC)	
Hematocrit	Male: 40-54% Female: 38-47%
Hemoglobin	Male: 13.5-18.0 gm/dl Female: 12.0-16.0 gm/dl
Red cell count	Male: 4.6-6.2 × 10^6/μl Female: 4.2-5.4 × 10^6/μl
White cell count	4500-11,000/μl
Erythrocyte indices	
Mean corpuscular volume (MCV)	82-98 cu microns (fl)
Mean corpuscular hemoglobin (MCH)	27-31 pg
Mean corpuscular hemoglobin concentration (MCHC)	32-36%

White blood cell differential (adult)

	Mean percent	Range of absolute counts
Segmented neutrophils	56%	(1800-7000/μl)
Bands	3%	(0-700/μl)
Eosinophils	2.7%	(0-450/μl)
Basophils	0.3%	(0-200/μl)
Lymphocytes	34%	(1000-4800/μl)
Monocytes	4%	(0-800/μl)

Test	Normal value
Blood volume	Male: 69 ml/kg Female: 65 ml/kg
Plasma volume	Male: 39 ml/kg Female: 40 ml/kg

Continued.

Table A-4. Hematology—cont'd

Test	Normal value
Coagulation tests	
Bleeding time (Ivy)	1-6 min
Bleeding time (Duke)	1-3 min
Clot retraction	½ the original mass in 2 hr
Dilute blood clot lysis time	Clot lyses between 6 and 10 hr at 37° C
Euglobin clot lysis time	Clot lyses between 2 and 6 hr at 37° C
Partial thromboplastin time (PTT)	60-70 sec
Kaolin activated	35-50 sec
Prothrombin time	12-14 sec
Venous clotting time	
3 tubes	5-15 min
2 tubes	5-8 min
Whole blood clot lysis time	None in 24 hr

Table A-5. Miscellaneous

Test	Specimen	Normal value
Bile, qualitative	Random stool	Negative in adults; positive in children
Chloride	Sweat	4-60 mEq/L
Clearances	Serum and timed urine	
Creatinine, endogenous		115 ± 20 ml/min
Diodrast		600-720 ml/min
Inulin		100-150 ml/min
PAH		600-750 ml/min
Diagnex blue (tubeless gastric analysis)	Urine	Free acid present
Fat	Stool, 72 hr	Total fat: <5 gm/24 hr and 10-25% of dry matter Neutral fat: 1-5% of dry matter Free fatty acids: 5-13% of dry matter Combined fatty acids: 5-15% of dry matter
Nitrogen, total	Stool, 24 hr	10% of intake or 1-2 gm/24 hr
Sodium	Sweat	10-80 mEq/L
Trypsin activity	Random, fresh stool	Positive (2 + to 4 +)
Thyroid ^{131}I uptake		7.5-25% in 6 hr
Urobilinogen		
Qualitative	Random stool	Positive
Quantitative	Stool, 24 hr	40-200 mg/24 hr 30-280 Ehrlich units/24 hr

Table A-6. Serology

Test	Normal value
Antibovine milk antibodies	Negative
Antideoxyribonuclease (ADNAase)	<1:20
Antinuclear antibodies (ANA)	<1:10
Antistreptococcal hyaluronidase (ASH)	<1:256
Antistreptolysin-O (ASLO)	<160 Todd units
Australia antigen	See hepatitis-associated antigen
Brucella agglutinins	<1:80
Coccidioidomycosis antibodies	Negative
Cold agglutinins	<1:32
Complement, C'3	100-170 mg/dl
C-reactive protein (CRP)	0
Fluorescent treponemal antibodies (FTA)	Nonreactive
Hepatitis-associated antigen (HAA or HBAg)	Negative
Heterophile antibodies	<1:56
Histoplasma agglutinins	<1:8
Latex fixation	Negative
Leptospira agglutinins	Negative
Ox cell hemolysin	<1:480
Rheumatoid factor	
Sensitized sheep cell	<1:160
Latex fixation	<1:80
Bentonite particles	<1:32
Streptococcal MG agglutinins	<1:20
Thyroid antibodies	
Antithyroglobulin	<1:32
Antithyroid microsomal	<1:56
Toxoplasma antibodies	<1:4
Trichina agglutinins	0
Tularemia agglutinins	<1:80
Typhoid agglutinins	
O	<1:80
H	<1:80
VDRL	Nonreactive
Weil-Felix (Proteus OX-2, OX-K, and OX-19 agglutinins)	Fourfold rise in titer between acute and convalescent sera

Table A-7. Cerebrospinal fluid

Test or constituent	Normal value	Special instructions
Albumin	10-30 mg/dl	
Albumin/globulin ratio	1.6-2.2	
Calcium	2.1-2.9 mEq/L	
Cell count	0-8 cells/μl	
Chloride	Adult: 118-132 mEq/L Children: 120-128 mEq/L	These values are invalidated by admixture of blood
Colloidal gold curve	0001111000	

Globulins
   Qualitative (Pandy)
   Quantitative
	
	 Negative
	 6-16 mg/dl	

Glucose	45-75 mg/dl	
Lactate dehydrogenase (LDH)	Approximately $^1/_{10}$ of serum level	

Protein
   Total CSF
   Ventricular fluid
	
	 15-45 mg/dl
	 8-15 mg/dl	

Protein electrophoresis
   Pre-albumin
   Albumin
   Alpha-1 globulin
   Alpha-2 globulin
   Beta globulin
   Gamma globulin
	
	 $4.1 \pm 1.2\%$
	 $62.4 \pm 5.6\%$
	 $5.3 \pm 1.2\%$
	 $8.2 \pm 2.0\%$
	 $12.8 \pm 2.0\%$
	 $7.2 \pm 1.1\%$	

Xanthochromia	Negative	

Normal values for echocardiographic examinations

The following tables represent normal values for echocardiographic examinations. The adult subjects were examined by Mrs. Sonia Chang between January, 1971 and March, 1972. The patients were examined in the supine and/or the left lateral positions. Except for the right ventricular dimension (RVD; see footnotes to Table B-1), the variation in position did not significantly influence the cardiac dimensions. Because of the changes in the right ventricular dimension, the measurements in both positions are listed. Less variation occurred in the supine RVD, and this is the preferred method of measuring this chamber. Dividing the cardiac chamber and aortic root measurements by the body surface area (Table B-2) narrows the range and provides more standardized values. Left ventricular wall thickness and aortic valve opening were not influenced significantly by body surface area and are not listed in Table B-2.

The children were examined by Dr. Lee Konecke between January, 1972 and June, 1972. All subjects were examined in the supine position. The values are arranged by both weight and body surface area. Grouping the data according to age did not prove useful.

Notes on tables: BSA = body surface area; RVD = right ventricular dimension between the anterior right ventricular wall and the right side of the interventricular septum at end-diastole; LVID = left ventricular internal dimension through the body of the left ventricle between the left side of the interventricular septum and the posterior left ventricular endocardium at end-diastole; left ventricular (LV) and interventricular (IV) septal wall thickness measured at end-diastole; left atrial (LA) dimension taken between the posterior aortic wall and the posterior left atrial wall at end-systole; aortic root = distance between the anterior and posterior aortic wall at the level of the aortic valve at end-diastole; aortic valve opening = separation of the aortic valve cusps with the onset of left ventricular ejection.

Reproduced with permission from Feigenbaum, H.: Echocardiography, Philadelphia, 1972, Lea and Febiger.

Table B-1. Normal adult values

	Mean	Range	Number of subjects
Age	27 yr	13-54 yr	75
BSA	1.79 M²	1.45-2.22 M²	74
RVD			
Supine	1.5 cm	0.7 -2.3 cm	39
Left lateral	1.7 cm	1.0 -2.6 cm	44
Change*	0.2 cm	0.0 -0.6 cm	8
LVID†	4.6 cm	3.5 -5.6 cm	73
LV wall thickness	0.9 cm	0.7 -1.1 cm	75
IV septal wall thickness	0.9 cm	0.7 -1.1 cm	73
LA dimension	2.9 cm	1.9 -4.0 cm	72
Aortic root	2.7 cm	2.0 -3.7 cm	64
Aortic valve opening	1.9 cm	1.6 -2.6 cm	44

*The change in RVD represents the difference between the supine and left lateral RVD measurements in eight subjects in whom both dimensions were obtained. Four additional subjects had marked increases in RVD (0.8-1.7 cm) when examined in the left lateral position, and their results are not included. This observation emphasizes why the examiner should rely on the supine RVD, especially if the left lateral RVD is enlarged.

†Three of the four subjects who had marked increases in left lateral RVD also decreased their LVID (0.8-1.3 cm). These subjects are not included. Although the change in LVID was less significant, one should be cautious about the left lateral LVID measurement if the left lateral RVD is abnormally large.

Table B-2. Normal adult values corrected for body surface area

	Mean (cm/M²)	Range (cm/M²)	Number of subjects
RVD			
Supine	0.9	0.5-1.2	38
Left lateral	0.9	0.4-1.3	44
LVID	2.6	1.9-3.2	73
LA	1.6	1.2-2.1	72
Aortic root	1.5	1.3-2.2	63

Table B-3. Normal values for children arranged by weight

	Weight (lbs)	Mean (cm)	Range (cm)	Number of subjects
RVD	0- 25	.9	.3-1.5	26
	26- 50	1.0	.4-1.5	26
	51- 75	1.1	.7-1.8	20
	76-100	1.2	.7-1.6	15
	101-125	1.3	.8-1.7	11
	126-200	1.3	1.2-1.7	5
LVID	0- 25	2.4	1.3-3.2	26
	26- 50	3.4	2.4-3.8	26
	51- 75	3.8	3.3-4.5	20
	76-100	4.1	3.5-4.7	15
	101-125	4.3	3.7-4.9	11
	126-200	4.9	4.4-5.2	5
LV and IV septal wall thickness	0- 25	.5	.4- .6	26
	26- 50	.6	.5- .7	26
	51- 75	.7	.6- .7	20
	76-100	.7	.7- .8	15
	101-125	.7	.7- .8	11
	126-200	.8	.7- .8	5
LA dimension	0- 25	1.7	.7-2.3	26
	26- 50	2.2	1.7-2.7	26
	51- 75	2.3	1.9-2.8	20
	76-100	2.4	2.0-3.0	15
	101-125	2.7	2.1-3.0	11
	126-200	2.8	2.1-3.7	5
Aortic root	0- 25	1.3	.7-1.7	26
	26- 50	1.7	1.3-2.2	26
	51- 75	2.0	1.7-2.3	20
	76-100	2.2	1.9-2.7	15
	101-125	2.3	1.7-2.7	11
	126-200	2.4	2.2-2.8	5
Aortic valve opening	0- 25	.9	.5-1.2	26
	26- 50	1.2	.9-1.6	26
	51- 75	1.4	1.2-1.7	20
	76-100	1.6	1.3-1.9	15
	101-125	1.7	1.4-2.0	11
	126-200	1.8	1.6-2.0	5

Table B-4. Normal values for children arranged by body surface area

	BSA (M²)	Mean (cm)	Range (cm)	Number of subjects
RVD	.5 or less	.8	.3-1.3	24
	.6 to 1.0	1.0	.4-1.8	39
	1.1 to 1.5	1.2	.7-1.7	29
	over 1.5	1.3	.8-1.7	11
LVID	.5 or less	2.4	1.3-3.2	24
	.6 to 1.0	3.4	2.4-4.2	39
	1.1 to 1.5	4.0	3.3-4.7	29
	over 1.5	4.7	4.2-5.2	11
LV and IV septal wall thickness	.5 or less	.5	.4- .6	24
	.6 to 1.0	.6	.5- .7	39
	1.1 to 1.5	.7	.6- .8	29
	over 1.5	.8	.7- .8	11
LA dimension	.5 or less	1.7	.7-2.4	24
	.6 to 1.0	2.1	1.8-2.8	39
	1.1 to 1.5	2.4	2.0-3.0	29
	over 1.5	2.8	2.1-3.7	11
Aortic root	.5 or less	1.2	.7-1.5	24
	.6 to 1.0	1.8	1.4-2.2	39
	1.1 to 1.5	2.2	1.7-2.7	29
	over 1.5	2.4	2.0-2.8	11
Aortic valve opening	.5 or less	.8	.5-1.0	24
	.6 to 1.0	1.3	.9-1.6	39
	1.1 to 1.5	1.6	1.3-1.9	29
	over 1.5	1.8	1.5-2.0	11

Normal values for cardiac catheterization

Table C-1. Normal values for pressures (at rest) in the cardiac chambers and vessels (mm Hg)

Location	Mean	Range
Right atrium		
Mean	2.8	1-5
a wave	5.6	2.5-7
z point	2.9	1-5.5
c wave	3.8	1.5-6
x' wave	1.7	0-5
v wave	4.6	2-7.5
y wave	2.4	0-6
Right ventricle		
Peak systolic	25	17-32
End-diastolic	4	1-7
Pulmonary artery		
Mean	15	9-19
Peak systolic	25	17-32
End-diastolic	9	4-13
Pulmonary artery wedge		
Mean	9	4-13
Left atrium		
Mean	7.9	2-12
a wave	10.4	4-16
z point	7.6	1-13
v wave	12.8	6-21
Left ventricle		
Peak systolic	130	90-140
End-diastolic	8.7	5-12
Brachial artery		
Mean	85	70-105
Peak systolic	130	90-140
End-diastolic	70	60-90

Table C-2. Normal values for cardiac output and related measurements

Measurements	Units	± SD
O_2 uptake	143 ml/min/m²	14.3
Arteriovenous O_2 difference	4.1 vol percent	0.6
Cardiac index	3.5 L/min/m²	0.7
Stroke index	46 ml/beat/m²	8.1

Table C-3. Oxygen content and saturation

Location	O_2 content vol %	O_2 saturation
Superior vena cava (SVC)	14 (±1)	70%
Inferior vena cave (IVC)	16 (±1)	80%
Right atrium (RA)	15 (±1)	75%
Pulmonary artery (PA)	15.2 (±1)	75%
Right ventricle (RV)	15.2 (±1)	75%
Brachial artery (BA)	19.0 (±1)	95%

Table C-4. Other measurements obtained during cardiac catheterization

$$\text{Pulmonary arteriolar resistance} = \frac{\text{Mean PA pressure} - \text{Mean PAW pressure (mm Hg)}}{\text{Pulmonary blood flow (L/min)}}$$

where:
$\qquad$ PA = Pulmonary artery

$\qquad$ PAW = Pulmonary artery wedge

Normal values for PAR = Less than 2.0 resistance units (less than 160 dynes sec cm^{-5})

$$\text{Total pulmonary resistance} = \frac{\text{Mean PA pressure} - \text{LV mean diastolic pressure (mm Hg)}}{\text{Pulmonary blood flow (L/min)}}$$

where:
$\qquad$ PA = Pulmonary artery

$\qquad$ LV = Left ventricle

Normal values for TPR = Less than 3.5 resistance units (less than 280 dynes see cm^{-5})

$$\text{Mitral valve area, } cm^2 = \frac{\text{Mitral valve flow (ml/sec)}}{31 \ \sqrt{\text{Diastolic gradient across the mitral valve}}}$$

where:
$\qquad$ $\text{Mitral valve flow} = \dfrac{\text{Cardiac output (ml/min)}}{\text{Diastolic filling period (sec/min)}}$

Diastolic filling period = Diastolic period per beat × Heart rate
(sec/min) $\qquad$ (sec/beat) $\qquad$ (beats/min)

Diastolic gradient across the = Left atrial mean pressure − Left ventricular mean diastolic
mitral valve (mm Hg) $\qquad$ (mm Hg) $\qquad$ pressure (mm Hg)

$\qquad$ 31 = Empirical constant

$$\text{Aortic valve area, } cm^2 = \frac{\text{Aortic valve flow (mo/sec)}}{44.5 \ \sqrt{\text{Systolic pressure gradient across the aortic valve}}}$$

where: $\qquad$ $\text{Aortic valve flow (mo/sec)} = \dfrac{\text{Cardiac output (ml/min)}}{\text{Systolic ejection period (sec/min)}}$

Systolic ejection period = Systolic ejection period per beat × Heart rate
(sec/min) $\qquad$ (sec/beat) $\qquad$ (beats/min)

Systolic pressure gradient across = Left ventricular mean systolid − Aortic mean systolic
the aortic valve (mm Hg) $\qquad$ pressure (mm Hg) $\qquad$ pressure (mm Hg)

$\qquad$ 44.5 = Gravity acceleration factor

$$\text{Cardiac output (L/min)} = \frac{I}{Ct} \times 60$$

where: I = Amount of indicator injected

$\qquad$ C = Mean concentration of indicator for the first circulation (mg/L)

$\qquad$ t = Time for the first circulation of indicator (seconds)

$$\text{Cardiac output (ml/min)} = \frac{\text{Oxygen consumption (ml/mm)}}{\text{Arterial } O_2 \text{ content} - \text{Mixed venous } O_2 \text{ content}} \times 100$$
$$\text{(vol \%)} \qquad\qquad \text{(vol \%)}$$

References

Anthony, C. P.: Textbook of anatomy and physiology, ed. 9, St. Louis, 1975, The C. V. Mosby Co.

Davidsohn, I., and Henry, J. B., editors: Todd-Sanford Clinical diagnosis by laboratory methods, ed. 15, Philadelphia, 1974, W. B. Saunders Co.

Feigenbaum, H., and Chang, S.: Echocardiography, Philadelphia, 1972, Lea & Febiger.

Felson, B.: Fundamentals of chest roentgenology, Philadelphia, 1973, W. B. Saunders Co.

Frankel, S., Reitman, S., Sonnenwirth, A. C., editors: Gradwohl's Clinical laboratory methods and diagnosis; a textbook on laboratory procedures and their interpretation, vols. I and II, ed. 7, St. Louis, 1970, The C. V. Mosby Co.

Harper, H. A.: Review of physiological chemistry, ed. 14, Los Altos, Calif., 1973, Lange Medical Publications.

Hurst, J. W., editor: The heart, ed. 3, New York, 1974, McGraw-Hill Book Co.

Mendel, D.: Practice of cardiac catheterization, ed. 2, Oxford, 1974, Blackwell Scientific Publications.

Ravel, R.: Clinical laboratory medicine: application of laboratory data, ed. 2, Chicago, 1973, Year Book Medical Publishers.

Schottelius, B. A., and Schottelius, D. D.: Textbook of physiology, ed. 17, St. Louis, 1973, The C. V. Mosby Co.

Slisenger, M. H., and Fordtran, J. S.: Gastrointestinal disease, pathophysiology, diagnosis, management, Philadelphia, 1973, W. B. Saunders Co.

Stollerman, G. H., editor: Advances in internal medicine, vols. 18 and 19, Chicago, 1972, Year Book Medical Publishers.

Tavell, M. E.: Clinical phonocardiography and external pulse recording, ed. 2, Chicago, 1972, Year Book Medical Publishers.

Weisler, A. M.: Noninvasive cardiology, New York, 1974, Grune & Stratton, Inc.

Wintrobe, et al, editors: Harrison's Principles of internal medicine, ed. 7, New York, 1974, McGraw-Hill Book Co.

Index

Boldface type indicates major discussion.

Electrocardiography
  ambulatory, 64-65
  in arrhythmias, 59-61
  in bundle branch block, 61
  and calcium, 5
  and CNS lesions, 58
  in congenital heart disease, 61
  in coronary artery disease, 57-58
  effects of drugs and electrolytes on, 61-63
  exercise, 65-67
  intracardiac, 60
  in second degree heart block, 60-61
  stress, 65-67
  in third degree heart block, 61
Electrocution and ventricular fibrillation, 60
Electroencephalogram, 174
Electrolytes, 17-28
  analysis explained, 17-18
  and arterial blood gases, 18
  and BUN, 18
  in congestive heart failure, 76
  and creatinine, 18
  disorder of, and ECG, 58, 60
  and ECG, 18, 61-63
  and pH, 18
  physiology of, 17
  specimen collection, 18-19
  and S-T depressions, 57
Electromyogram, 175
Electrophoresis, protein, 12
  hemoglobin, 164
  and hypocalcemia, 4
  and LDH, 14
  and lipoproteins, 75
  and macroglobulinemia, 12
  and multiple myeloma, 12
  normal values
    CSF, 204
    serum, 190
  and reversed A/G ratio, 12
Electroshock therapy and neutrophilic leukocytosis, 28
Embden-Meyerhof pathway, 166
Emboli, pulmonary, 105
  and angiography, 88
  and heparin, 77
  and LDH, 15, 43
  and lung scan, 85
  and pulmonary angiography, 101
  and pulmonary perfusion scan, 100
  tests for, 105
EMG; *see* Electromyogram
Emphysema, differential diagnosis of, 102
Endocardial cushion defect, and ECG, 61
Endocarditis
  infective, 77-78
  subacute bacterial, and acute glomerulonephritis, 115
Endocrine system
  anatomy and physiology of (general), 143
  tests for disorders, 141-158
Endomyocardium, small vessel disease of, 91

Endoscopy, 120
Enteritis
  acute radiation, 129
  eosinophilic, 129
  regional, 129, **131**
Enteropathy, protein losing, 29
Enzyme assays, erythrocyte, 165
Enzyme deficiency and hypocholesterolemia, 11
Enzymes, 12-16
  cardiac, 73-75
    clinical value of, 75
  physiology of, 12-13
Eosinopenia, **27**, 48
Eosinophilia, on peripheral smear, 32
Eosinophilic enteritis, 129
Eosinophilic leukocytosis, **28**, 48
Eosinophilic pneumonias, 106
Eosinophils, 20, **25-26**, 48
  normal value, 201
Epileptic lesions and EEG, 174
Epinephrine, 150
  normal urine, 197
Erythrocyte indices, 30-32
  normal values, 201
Erythropoietin, 30, 31
Esophageal spasm, diffuse, 123
  differential diagnosis, **123**, 124
  tests for, 123
Esophagitis, differential diagnosis, and tests for, 123
Esophagoscopy with biopsy, 123, 124
Esophagus
  acidity test, **122**, 123
  anatomy and physiology of, 122
  laboratory tests, 122-124
  rupture of, 124
ESR; *see* Sedimentation rate
Estrogens
  and hypokalemia, 21
  normal urine, 197
Etiocholanolone, normal urine, 198
Extrasystoles, 59-60
Extrinsic factor, 129
Exudates, 100

F

Fanconi syndrome; *see* De Fanconi
Fat
  neutral, normal serum, 193
  normal stool, 128, 202
Fats, normal blood, 190
Fatty acids, normal blood, 190
Favism, 165
Fecal fat content, 128, 202
Fecal urobilinogen
  in jaundice, 136, 137
  normal, 135, 136, 202
Felty's syndrome, 27
"Fetal" alpha₁ globulin, 140
FEV₁; *see* Forced expiratory volume
FEV/VC%, **98**, 102
Fever
  and elevated BUN, 17